TREATING SOMATIZATION

TREATING SOMATIZATION

A Cognitive-Behavioral Approach

Robert L. Woolfolk
Lesley A. Allen

THE GUILFORD PRESS
New York   London

© 2007 The Guilford Press
A Division of Guilford Publications, Inc.
72 Spring Street, New York, NY 10012
www.guilford.com

Printed in the United States of America

This book is printed on acid-free paper.

Last digit is print number: 9   8   7   6   5   4   3   2   1

Library of Congress Cataloging-in-Publication Data

Woolfolk, Robert L.
  Treating somatization : a cognitive-behavioral approach / by Robert L. Woolfolk and Lesley A. Allen.
      p. ; cm.
  Includes bibliographical references and index.
  ISBN-10: 1-59385-350-5   ISBN-13: 978-1-59385-350-1 (hardcover : alk. paper)
  1. Somatization disorder.   2. Medicine, Psychosomatic.   3. Cognitive therapy.   I. Allen, Lesley A.   II. Title.
  [DNLM: 1. Somatoform Disorders—therapy.   2. Cognitive Therapy—methods. WM 170 W913t 2006]
  RC552.S66W662 2006
  616.85′24—dc22

                                                                          2006012304

To Katie

About the Authors

Robert L. Woolfolk, PhD, is Professor of Psychology and Philosophy at Rutgers University and Visiting Professor of Psychology at Princeton University. He has published many papers and several books on psychotherapy and psychopathology, including *Stress, Sanity, and Survival* (1978, Monarch) and *The Cure of Souls: Science, Values, and Psychotherapy* (1998, Jossey-Bass). A practicing clinician for more than 30 years, Dr. Woolfolk has sought in both his work with patients and his scholarly endeavors to integrate the scientific and humanistic traditions of psychotherapy.

Lesley A. Allen, PhD, is a clinical psychologist and Associate Professor of Psychiatry at Robert Wood Johnson Medical School at the University of Medicine and Dentistry of New Jersey. She has authored or coauthored numerous journal articles and book chapters on somatoform disorders. Dr. Allen is actively involved in clinical work, teaching, and supervising. She is currently Principal Investigator on an ongoing program of clinical research funded by the National Institute of Mental Health.

Acknowledgments

Writing any book entails a variety of struggles that are successful only with the assistance of others. We owe thanks to several people. Mike Gara provided theoretical and methodological guidance, sound practical judgment, and occasional flashes of brilliance. Paul Lehrer was there at the beginning with his unsurpassed scholarship and estimable clinical wisdom. Javier Escobar's enlightened administrative leadership and impeccable intellectual sensibilities were indispensable to the project. Jim Nageotte of The Guilford Press provided the optimal combination of encouragement and oversight. Thanks also to Seymour Weingarten for being everything a publisher should be.

We owe our deepest gratitude, however, to the many patients and trainees who have labored along with us to alleviate the form of suffering that this book addresses.

The writing of this book and the research described herein were partially supported by grants from the National Institute of Mental Health (Grant Nos. K08 MH01662, R21 MH066831, R01 MH60265, and P20 MH074634).

Contents

TREATING SOMATIZATION

Introduction

Somatization is among the most puzzling phenomena that health-care workers encounter. In somatization physical symptoms occur in the absence of any identifiable causal mechanism. The causes of somatization that we are able to implicate are neither proximate nor somatic, seeming instead to be indirect and to reside in the patient's mind or culture. Somatization appears to be universal. We find it in all present societies and in all past societies for which we have relevant records. Forty centuries ago, the physicians of Egypt were familiar with somatization; some years later so were those of ancient Greece.

For the contemporary clinician, the patient who somatizes is a pressing practical problem. Here there is distress, dysfunction, and disability of great magnitude and intransigence. Patients diagnosed with the most severe form of somatization, somatization disorder, have been shown to incur healthcare expenses that are nine times the U.S. average and consume disproportionate amounts of the time and energy of healthcare providers (Smith, Monson, & Ray, 1986a). In addition to the extensive direct costs, somatization disorder creates enormous indirect costs to the economy in the form of lost work productivity. Individuals diagnosed with somatization disorder report being bedridden for 2–7 days per month (Katon et al., 1991; Smith et al., 1986a). Somatization disorder is not only costly, but also difficult to treat successfully. In a longitudinal study following patients with somatization disorder who were receiving standard medical care, only 31% recovered after 15 years (Coryell & Norten, 1981). Typically, patients with somatization disorder are dissatisfied with the medical services they receive and repeatedly change physicians (Lin et al.,

1991). These "treatment-resistant" patients frustrate healthcare providers with their frequent complaints and dissatisfaction with treatment (Lin et al., 1991). No controlled medication trial for somatization disorder has been published. Anecdotal evidence suggests that many patients diagnosed with somatization disorder refuse to take medication and that those who do frequently report adverse medication side effects (Murphy, 1982). The story is much the same with other polysymptomatic somatoform disorders (Fallon, 2004). As of this writing, pharmacological treatment has had minimal success with somatization.

In this book we describe our efforts to alleviate the suffering of patients with somatization. Over the last decade, we have developed a dedicated psychosocial treatment for somatization that draws upon various traditions in psychotherapy, especially cognitive-behavioral therapy and emotion-focused experiential therapies, a treatment we call affective cognitive-behavioral therapy (ACBT). The principal aim of this book is to describe that treatment and to provide the training material necessary for its effective use. To frame our approach to this problem, we first provide a brief review of the history of somatization and of psychosomatic medicine. We then discuss philosophical and sociocultural underpinnings of somatization and conclude with an overview of theories of somatization.

BACKGROUND: HISTORICAL AND THEORETICAL

The history of somatization begins with hysteria. Hysteria was first described 4,000 years ago by the Egyptians. Typical cases involved pain in the absence of any injury or pathology in the location of the pain. The Egyptian theory held that a wandering uterus moved about the body and produced pain from various regions. Greek physicians described a similar set of psychosomatic symptoms and essentially retained the Egyptian theory. The Greeks gave us the word *hysteria*, from the Greek *hystera*, meaning womb. The Greco-Egyptian formulation reveals two noteworthy features: that the disorder was primarily observed in females and that there was something thought to be essentially female about the disorder. Although the diagnostic category subsumed more than somatization, the term hysteria continued to be widely used to label somatization patients until 30 years ago.

Medieval and Renaissance medicine preserved the ancient formulation of hysteria as described by the ultimate authorities, Hippocrates and Galen, until the 17th and 18th centuries, when it was first linked with the nervous system and the emotions. At the beginning of the

17th century, the French physician Charles Le Pois opposed the uterine theory of hysteria (he believed the spleen to be the culprit) and declared that hysteria could occur in men; a few years later, Thomas Sydenham declared that hysteria was the result of psychological and emotional causes and that in men hysteria was manifested as hypochondria (Boss, 1979). Foucault (1961/1965) states that by the end of the 18th century hysteria and hypochondria were beginning to be viewed as diseases of the nerves akin to such recognized mental disorders as melancholia. By the 18th century, some authorities, such as Joseph Raulin, began to question hysteria's organic basis. Raulin described hysteria as a "disease in which women invent, exaggerate, and repeat all the various absurdities of which a disordered imagination is capable" (quoted in Foucault, 1961/1965, pp. 137–138). Before the 19th century, due to the heterogeneous nature of hysterical symptoms and the hypothesized connection with the emotions, physicians had begun to allege that these symptoms were feigned or imagined. The unsympathetic attitudes of contemporary healthcare workers toward somatizers and the tendency to regard them as malingerers can be traced to this period in the history of medicine.

Paul Briquet's (1859) seminal monograph, *Traité Clinique et Thérapeutique de L'hystérie*, was a landmark in the descriptive psychopathology of somatization. Our current conception of somatization disorder derives directly from this paper. Briquet's meticulous and exhaustive listing of the symptomatology of hysteria remains unsurpassed. In fact, he described three related syndromes: conversion phenomena, hysterical personality, and multiple chronic unexplained somatic symptoms (Dongier, 1983; Mai & Merskey, 1980), all overlapping in symptomatology somewhat and often observed to co-occur. Briquet's perspicuous work was revived by Purtell, Robins, and Cohen (1951) and developed further by members of the illustrious Washington University Department of Psychiatry. Perley and Guze (1962) published a list of 57 symptoms commonly reported by women diagnosed with hysteria, symptoms that were clustered in 10 different areas. These investigators were the first to suggest specific criteria for the diagnosis of hysteria: the presence of 25 symptoms from at least 9 of the 10 symptom areas (Guze, 1967). Later, this list of 57 symptoms was expanded to 59 symptoms and the term "Briquet's syndrome" was adopted (Guze, Woodruff, & Clayton, 1972). The criteria for Briquet's syndrome were incorporated into the Feighner criteria (Feighner et al., 1972), the precursor to the symptom set that appeared in the third edition of the *Diagnostic and Statistical Manual of Mental Disorders* (DSM-III; American Psychiatric Association, 1980). In that volume the theoretically neutral term "somatization" was preferred over the traditional terminology.

Although some of the traditional language remains in the fourth edition of the DSM (e.g., "conversion disorder"), the word "hysteria" no longer appears (DSM-IV; American Psychiatric Association, 1994). The ninth edition of the World Health Organization's (1979) *International Classification of Diseases* (ICD-9), a more cosmopolitan nosology of somatic and mental disorders published a year earlier than DSM-III, retains much of the perennial terminology, including not only hysteria but also "neurasthenia."[1] ICD-10 (World Health Organization, 1993) has shifted in the direction of the DSM, though without banishing every bit of the classical vocabulary.

The history of somatization also is interconnected with two important and historically related developments in the history of psychiatry: (1) psychosomatic medicine and (2) psychoanalysis. Although eventually absorbed by psychoanalysis and subsumed within a psychoanalytic theoretical framework, psychosomatic medicine had an established history before Freud. From antiquity, the interaction between mind and body and its effects upon health had been alluded to by many writers. An early systematic account was William Falconer's (1788) *A Dissertation on the Influence of the Passions upon the Disorders of the Body*. The term "psychosomatic" was used first by Heinroth in 1818 as "describing the interplay between mind and body in health and disease" (West, 1982, p. xvi). By the end of the 19th century "nervous conditions," including psychosomatic ailments such as neurasthenia, and the "nerve doctors" who treated them had proliferated, so much so that during the Victorian era "bad nerves" was thought of as something of an epidemic (Shorter, 1997).

It was about this time that Sigmund Freud entered upon the scene. As a young man Freud spent the winter of 1885–86 as a student of Jean-Martin Charcot at the Salpêtrière hospital in Paris. There he observed the world's leading authority, Charcot, use hypnosis to remove hysterical symptoms. Upon his return to Vienna, Freud began a close collaboration with Joseph Breuer. The product of this collaboration was the book *Studies in Hysteria* (1895/1974), in which Breuer and Freud developed the concept of "conversion," a process whereby intrapsychic activity putatively brings about somatic symptoms. Although Freud was later to break with Breuer and go on to create the substan-

---

[1]Neurasthenia is defined in ICD-10 as persistent and distressing feelings of exhaustion after minor mental or physical effort, accompanied by one or more of the following symptoms: muscular aches or pains, dizziness, tension headache, sleep disturbance, inability to relax, and irritability. The term was coined in 1856 by Robert Mayne and popularized by the American neurologist George Beard during the second half of the 19th century (Gijswijt-Hofstra & Porter, 2001).

tial edifice of psychoanalysis, his work on hysteria was a blueprint for and harbinger of later theoretical efforts. Here the ideas of early emotional trauma or intrapsychic conflict as the cause of physical symptoms began to take shape. This work also introduced the notion of a physical symptom as an unconscious form of communication, a device for securing secondary gain, or a means for avoiding emotional pain.

The notion of the transduction of psychological conflict into bodily symptoms was widely disseminated as psychoanalysis began to dominate psychiatry. Stekel (1924) coined the term "somatization" (*somatisieren*) during the early 1920s and defined it as "the conversion of emotional states into physical symptoms" (p. 341). That is, Stekel regarded somatization as equivalent to the mechanism of conversion that Breuer and Freud had used to explain the development of sensory or voluntary motor symptoms in hysteria. A strident and eccentric proponent of the mind–body interaction was Georg Groddeck (1977), who believed that psychic processes are etiological factors in all diseases (Avila & Winston, 2003). Groddeck contended that the symptoms of any somatic disease might be interpreted as symbolic expressions of unconscious motives and caused via the same mechanisms believed to underlie hysteria.

The father of modern American psychosomatic medicine, Franz Alexander, attempted to minimize the excesses of indiscriminate psychoanalytic approaches such as Groddeck's. Alexander (1950) took great pains to distinguish between two types of psychosomatic symptoms: (1) those cases in which psychological conflict was "converted" and communicated symbolically through physical symptoms, and (2) those cases in which the somatic symptoms resulted from the direct and indirect physiological effects of emotional arousal. This second kind of psychosomatic mechanism required few, if any, psychoanalytic assumptions and was quite compatible with mainstream scientific research, especially the work of Cannon, Seyle, and others on psychosocial stress. As psychoanalysis declined in influence, psychosomatic medicine declined also. Today, the term "psychosomatic," which was faddish in the 1950s, is no longer in vogue. Many of the problems once treated within the context of psychosomatic medicine now fall under the purview of what is, in some sense, its successor discipline: behavioral medicine.

SOCIOCULTURAL AND PHILOSOPHICAL ISSUES

The biopsychosocial concept of illness, proposed by George Engel (1977) and to which we subscribe, suggests that illness is a complex entity involving the interplay of physical, psychological, and cultural factors. In particular, many illnesses cannot be adequately comprehended without taking into account the social contexts in which they develop and are manifested, diagnosed, and treated. What phenomena societies come to label illness or how human suffering is expressed and presented to healers are complicated matters that can be conceptualized at several different levels, levels that involve variables that interact causally. The advent of such disciplines as psychoneuroimmunology and behavioral medicine has brought us evidence, in many domains of medicine, of the close connections and complex concurrent interactions among mental, behavioral, and somatic variables. When we examine many somatic illnesses (e.g., hypertension) from the various standpoints of etiology, symptomatology, and treatment, they emerge as complex entities with multifaceted interacting components, with biological, psychological, and social causes (Baum & Posluszny, 1999; Cohen & Herbert, 1996). In the case of mental disorders or psychiatric syndromes the situation is even more complex and the levels of explanation more deeply intertwined.

The historical record shows that Western categories of psychopathology have been influenced strongly by sociocultural factors and that what gets labeled a mental illness is, to some degree, a reflection of cultural values. Drapetomania, the desire of slaves to escape captivity, was in the early 19th century considered a mental illness (Cartwright, 1851/1981; Szasz, 1987). Victorian physicians regularly performed "therapeutic" clitorectomies on masturbators, who were thought to be mentally ill. As recently as 1938, listed among the 40 psychiatric disorders in a leading textbook (Rosanoff, 1938) were moral deficiency, masturbation, misanthropy, and vagabondage. Homosexuality, which Western psychiatry regarded as a manifestation of mental illness, was "officially" depathologized, after a contentious political struggle, by a referendum of the American Psychiatric Association membership in 1974 (Kutchins & Kirk, 1997). Not so long ago, psychiatrists in the former Soviet Union performed the Orwellian maneuver of medicalizing opposition to the state when they employed the diagnosis of "sluggish schizophrenia" to effect the incarceration of many political dissidents (Bloch & Reddaway, 1977). Symptoms that indicate pathology in one society (e.g., regularly hearing the voice of a dead relative) are normal and customary in others.

Cultural variation in psychopathology results not only from differences in how psychiatric labels are applied, but from the fact that different societies seem to produce different forms of psychopathology. Many specific syndromes are unique to particular cultural contexts, such as *ataque de nervios, koro,* or *taijin kyofusho.*[2] The epidemics of anorexia nervosa and bulimia in the contemporary West are unprecedented but are spreading to middle and upper classes around the world along with Westernization and its current aesthetic ideal of a slender female body (Ung & Lee, 1999). Writers such as Ian Hacking (1995, 1999) have argued persuasively that some mental disorders (e.g., multiple personality disorder) consist of roles that are created by the theories and practices of the mental health professions and subsequently enacted by patients. The articulation and dissemination of information about psychopathology through professional activities and by the media provide a symptom set and patient profile that can be assimilated by disturbed individuals who possess sufficient psychic malleability (Woolfolk, 1998).

Historically in Western psychiatry, a mental disorder has been posited in one of two instances. The first of these occurs when there exists a theory of psychogenesis, such as psychoanalysis, that hypothesizes mental entities to be the underlying causes of the symptoms of a disorder. The second instance involves the presence of symptoms in the absence of a physicalistic explanation. In this second instance, psychogenic etiology may be inferred solely from the absence of a known underlying physical mechanism, thus revealing a tacit dualism that originated even before Paracelsus and that continues to underlie Western medicine: Disease entities, whether they be causes or symptoms, belong to one of two categories, either the physical or the mental, these two categories being mutually exclusive (Robinson, 1996). Symptoms of almost any variety that cannot be linked to a scientifically explained physical pathology are assumed to be psychogenic. Individuals afflicted with multiple sclerosis, Wilson's disease, temporal lobe epilepsy, and numerous other maladies currently within the purview of somatic medicine were once regarded as mentally ill. Through the course of medical progress, mental illness has served as a residual category wherein poorly understood or refractory illness has been placed, often temporarily, only to be removed when medical science established the physical mechanisms underlying the disorder (Grob, 1991).

Dualistic assumptions operate not so subtly within DSM-IV. In DSM-IV two principal classes of disease entities are posited: (1) general medical conditions and (2) primary mental disorders. Contradistinct from the most paradigmatic mental disorders contained in DSM-IV are mental symptoms resulting from a "general medical con-

---

[2]Each of these "culture-specific syndromes" comprises somatic and psychological symptoms.

dition" (read: physical illness). Symptoms arising from such causes, indeed, imply the absence of a mental disorder. Of course, DSM-IV's authors claim that the distinction between primary mental disorders and those stemming from a general medical condition should not be taken to imply that there are fundamental differences between mental disorders and general medical conditions (American Psychiatric Association, 1994, p. 165). But the volume is careful to distinguish symptoms deriving from a general medical disorder from those that emanate from a primary mental disorder. This distinction is drawn so sharply that symptoms of organic origin are exclusionary for the diagnosis of such paradigmatic disorders as schizophrenia. The locution of the volume instantiates not only dualism, but also logical circularity, in that a general medical condition is defined as a medical condition other than a primary mental disorder, and a primary mental disorder is defined as something other than the result of a general medical condition. The distinction drawn here, whether nominal or substantive, is old Cartesian wine in a new bottle, that venerable distinction between the functional and the organic. In its language DSM-IV also stipulates, as a kind of axiom, the historical role of psychiatry as a processor of aberrations within the category of illness. Mental illnesses are abnormal, poorly understood illnesses that normal physicians do not treat.

Some have argued that the concept of somatization is unintelligible in medical traditions without a dualistic ontology. In many societies the concept of somatization has no meaning, since distinctions between mental and physical illness are not prevalent (Fabrega, 1991). For example, within the medical traditions of China and India, illness is conceived holistically in terms of various imbalances. The mind–body distinction is neither fundamental nor sharply drawn.

Studies of mental illness in non-Western societies reveal that somatic, rather than psychological symptomatology, often is the primary indication of a psychiatric disorder. For example, research in China has found that symptoms of psychiatric patients were predominantly somatic. For years the most commonly diagnosed mental disorder in China has been *shenjing shuairuo*, an indigenous diagnostic category signifying a "weakness of nerves" (Parker, Gladstone, & Chee, 2001). This disorder is described in the *Chinese Classification of Mental Diseases, 2nd Edition, Revised* (CCMD-2-R; Chinese Medical Association & Nanjing Medical University, 1995) and is accepted as a commonplace and legitimate illness by both medical practitioners and the general public. The disorder, oddly enough, is characterized largely by somatic symptoms, many of the same symptoms treated by Euroamerican "nerve doctors" in the 19th century, such as fatigue (Shorter, 1997).

Hence, the disorder is most often translated for Westerners as neurasthenia. Medical anthropologist Arthur Kleinman (1982) evaluated a sample of Chinese neurasthenics and determined that the majority manifested significant depressive symptomatology, albeit not sufficient nor in the requisite configuration to meet DSM criteria for a diagnosis of major depression. He concluded that many Chinese given the neurasthenia diagnosis could be suffering from depression, though not the Euroamerican form of depression that is characterized by despondence and patterns of thinking described by cognitive theorists such as Aaron Beck (Beck, 1976; Beck, Rush, Shaw, & Emery, 1979). In fact, studies of depression in China have found that relatively few Chinese manifest the DSM-IV syndrome of depressed mood, self-criticism, guilt, and pessimism. Chinese epidemiological research also suggests that patients with anxiety, like patients with depression, present a greater ratio of somatic to psychological symptoms than that found in the West (Parker, Cheah, & Roy, 2001; Tsoi, 1985; Zhang, Shen, & Li, 1998).

Research on psychopathology in China frequently is used to argue that cultural factors are crucial in determining the manner in which human suffering is experienced and, more specifically, to support the view that non-Western societies are prone to generate somatic expressions of distress. One distinction that is made in cross-cultural theory is that between somatization and "psychologization." The former refers to the experience of bodily aspects of distress whereas the latter refers to the experience of the psychic, social, and mental aspects of distress (Kirmayer, 1984; White, 1982). According to this formulation, either somatization or psychologization could serve as alternative modalities through which a negative emotional reaction is experienced and as alternative "idioms of distress" through which emotional pain is communicated. It has been suggested that psychologization is compatible with Western, Euroamerican concepts of selfhood and with an individualistic, psychologically minded worldview that emphasizes causal explanations implicating individuals and their traits as sources of events (Kihlstrom & Canter Kihlstrom, 1999; Kirmayer, Young, & Robbins, 1994). Somatization, in contrast, has been associated with the more sociocentric cultural views of selfhood where self-reflection and self-examination are deemphasized or disvalued; here, behavior is more often viewed as caused by the external environment, rather than by qualities of the person such as psychological traits or willpower. Other factors that might influence the ratio of psychologization to somatization are the stigma attached to psychological symptoms and the degree to which a desired treatment is obtained through either a psychological or a somatic presentation (Kirmayer, 2001).

The twin, reciprocal processes of somatization and psychologization are at first glance somewhat obscure and inaccessible. The workings are most often illustrated by examples of how emotional distress might be somatized. But let us first take the example of how a physical illness might be psychologized. Suppose you are a person who has contracted a mild viral infection and you are beginning to become symptomatic. Typically, if you conduct an examination of your initial symptoms, you may tend to emphasize elevated core body temperature or gastrointestinal motility, which you or your healthcare provider can readily link to the effect of a viral infection. The most familiar bodily discomforts of an infection constitute an incomplete inventory of all of its adverse accompaniments. There may be feelings of lethargy and dysphoria and difficulty concentrating. Why emphasize the former somatic symptomatology rather than the latter "psychological" effects of an infection? One could argue that the practice depends upon the patient's frame of reference. We report our physical symptoms, it could be argued, because we think we have an illness, which we conceive as a disorder stemming from physical causes, the important effects of and treatments for we believe to be somatic. Yet suppose you have the aforementioned symptoms but do not know that you have an infection and do not, therefore, privilege and adopt a physicalistic frame of reference. Suppose, also, that you are in the midst of a psychological crisis, such as job loss or divorce. Perhaps you have recently seen a daytime television talk show on which people report the various adverse emotional effects of psychological stress. Under these circumstances, with an attributional bias primed by salient psychosocial perturbations, you might be less inclined to measure your body temperature and, instead, might be disposed to focus on your mental state and conclude that you are depressed or "stressed out."

The theory we have been describing assumes that the background assumptions or the "idiom of distress" is crucial to determining whether a disruption of homeostasis is experienced as physical or mental. An individual can learn to attend to and express physical discomfort, rather than psychological distress, especially if an idiom of affect is not available. Thus, the theory has it that somatization conditions can be shaped through processes of selective attention to physical symptoms and by learning a vocabulary of somatic symptomatology.

Part of the allure of cross-cultural research on somatization symptoms is the possibility that cultural differences in the experience of illness might hold the key to understanding the mechanisms that underlie somatization. At this juncture, however, cross-cultural research on unexplained physical symptoms must be regarded as inconclusive and fraught with methodological problems, including confounds involving socioeconomic factors and cross-cultural differences in healthcare systems.

Whether there are cultures that foster somatization is still a complex and controversial question. The World Health Organization's international collaborative study of Psychological Problems in General Health Care (Gureje, Simon, Ustun, & Goldberg, 1997) did not find the disparity in somatization disorders between East and West that might have been predicted from the early formulations of medical anthropologists. Nor did the ratio of somatic to psychological symptoms of depression vary across cultures in a systematic or expected fashion. The data were, however, to some degree consistent with the cultural hypothesis. For example, somatization rates were significantly higher in Latin America than in the rest of the world, and rates of somatization were higher in China than in the United States (Simon, Von Korff, Piccinelli, Fullerton, & Ormel, 1999). This study failed to include indigenous, culture-specific syndromes or to analyze single-symptom presentations, nor was there adequate assessment of the ratio of somatization to psychologization in the more frequently diagnosed forms of psychopathology, such as depression. A study that provides probative evidence on relative somatizing versus psychologizing tendencies across cultures has yet to be conducted.

MODELS OF SOMATIZATION

Not since the psychoanalytic era has somatization been viewed as a well-understood phenomenon. In some sense we have not progressed very far beyond Breuer and Freud's psychodynamic theory of conversion hysteria. Currently, there is widespread admission among authorities that no adequate theory of somatization exists. Indeed, one might argue that, with the exception of the oft-criticized and scientifically beleaguered psychoanalytic theory, there are no well-developed theories of somatization, only some fragmentary models or speculation. In Chapter 3, we describe and analyze some models of somatization and examine the relevant empirical evidence supporting each.

In evaluating models of somatization one needs to be mindful of the logical pitfalls that abound in the territory of mind–body relationships. As we have seen in conjecture about the cause of somatization, such phrases as "emotional distress expressed as physical symptoms" or a "somatic idiom of distress" or a tendency to "somatize rather than

psychologize" are invoked. Such locutions are problematic and bespeak the poverty of our theories as they invariably risk the possibility
of emerging as either pseudoexplanatory or tautologous. Such formulations often fail to explain because they leave key terms undefined
and unexplicated. We have seen this kind of fallacious logic before in
psychiatric discourse that utilizes the notion of "chemical imbalance"
in explanations of the treatment of depression—that is, a prior chemical imbalance is inferred from a presumptive "balancing" of neuro-
chemistry by antidepressants. Key concepts that are unexplained can
result in circular reasoning, illustrated by Moliere's physician who
attributed the effect of a soporific to its "dormative powers." A cogent
explanation of somatization must spell out exactly what is denoted by
the "emotional distress" that is putatively "expressed" somatically and
also include valid and reliable methods for measuring it. Can the emotional distress thought to underlie somatization be identified indepen-
dently of its somatic expression? If not, what is the epistemological status of our model or theory? Are we simply assuming a priori that there
is some emotional basis for any unexplained physical symptom? If so,
we have engaged in question begging rather than explanation.

Fortunately for scientists, healthcare providers, and patients, various diagnoses and the forms of psychotherapy and pharmacotherapy
applied are warranted, for the most part, by empirical findings that
validate clinical practices rather than confirm underlying theory. There
are few cases in psychiatry in which a treatment can be shown to produce clinical benefits because it affects a well-understood mechanism
that is implicated conclusively in pathogenesis. We simply do not have
theories or models of mental disorders that have been validated in the
manner of our theories of, for example, infectious diseases. Our technologies of healing are legitimized not by the verification of the underlying theory, but by the efficacies of these technologies. Research on
treatments for mental disorders is much more akin to industrial practices of product testing than to theory-based applied science. Fortunately, effective clinical interventions need not wait upon validated scientific theories of psychiatric disorder. We and our colleagues, as did
the empirics of old, put our money on pragmatic observable results of
interventions, as opposed to armchair speculation about the true
nature of things.

This is not to say that we practice "dust-bowl" empiricism or are
unguided or undisciplined by a priori assumptions, models, and theories. Our approach to somatization draws heavily on several sources:
(1) stress research and the stress-management and self-regulation
literature; (2) the contemporary psychology of emotion and those

experiential approaches to psychotherapy that emphasize emotional processing; (3) social learning theory and the cognitive-behavioral interventions that are predicated on cognitive-appraisal and conditioning models of behavior; (4) role theory as it derives from sociocultural analyses of illness behavior by sociologists and medical anthropologists. In Chapter 3, we elaborate the rationale for our treatment, but first, in Chapter 2, we define more precisely the problem we wish to treat.

Somatization

Epidemiology, Clinical Characteristics, and Treatment

Maria had just lifted the last bag of groceries out of her shopping cart. As she turned toward the open hatch of her SUV, a sharp, stabbing pain made her cry out. As she clutched her lower abdomen, the bag landed on the pavement and its contents spilled out onto the parking lot. Out of the corner of her eye, Maria saw an orange rolling rapidly away from her. She cursed quietly as she realized that she was doubled over with a searing pain that ran between her hips and across the front of her body. Slowly, Maria lowered herself to the pavement and lay on her side. She had experienced this pain before and knew that if she reclined, it would eventually subside. The pains had begun in her late 20s, and doctors had been of little help. Irritable bowel syndrome was the diagnosis that the gastroenterologist had given her. Maria had tried various treatments, without any real benefit. Her primary care physician had suggested that stress was the likely cause, but that conjecture had not been helpful. Maria tried to reduce her stress, but the pains seemed unpredictable and unrelated to other events in her life. They would come, out of the blue, even when she felt calm.

Our treatment is designed for patients with multiple unexplained physical symptoms, including both patients who meet full criteria for somatization disorder and those whose symptoms are not sufficiently numerous or diverse to qualify for a somatization disorder diagnosis. We have adopted this broad definition of somatization because it seems to reside on a continuum, one that cannot be adequately represented by a categorical scheme (Katon et al., 1991). We would suggest that somatization disorder represents one extreme on the somatization continuum and that subthreshold somatization (including undifferentiated somatoform disorder, multisomatoform disorder, abridged somatization, irritable bowel syndrome, chronic fatigue syndrome, and fibromyalgia) lies closer to the midpoint on the same continuum.

This chapter reviews the diagnostic criteria for the aforementioned somatization-spectrum disorders, as well as the epidemiology, clinical characteristics, and treatments associated with the various disorders.

DEFINITIONS AND EPIDEMIOLOGY

Somatization Disorder

Although medicine has long recognized the existence of a group of patients with multiple medically unexplained symptoms and abnormal illness behavior, there has been and continues to be disagreement over the precise diagnostic criteria for somatization disorder. The term *somatization disorder* was introduced in the third edition of the American Psychiatric Association's classification system, the *Diagnostic and Statistical Manual of Mental Disorders* (DSM-III; American Psychiatric Association, 1980). The criteria required for its diagnosis have been revised in each of the manual's subsequent versions. According to DSM-III, somatization disorder in men is characterized by a lifetime history of at least 12 medically unexplained physical symptoms; for women, the diagnosis requires a history of at least 14 medically unexplained physical symptoms (American Psychiatric Association, 1980). Abandoning DSM-III's gender distinction, DSM-III-R defines somatization disorder as a lifetime history of at least 13 medically unexplained physical symptoms for both men and women (American Psychiatric Association, 1987). More recently, the authors of DSM-IV reduced the number of symptoms required for the somatization disorder diagnosis to eight, while introducing the requirement that those symptoms involve multiple bodily systems. According to DSM-IV (American Psychiatric Association, 1994), somatization disorder is characterized by at least four unexplained pain symptoms, two unexplained non-pain gastrointestinal symptoms, one unexplained sexual or menstrual symptom, and one pseudoneurological symptom (see Table 2.1). The World Health Organization (WHO) has offered yet another set of diagnostic criteria for somatization disorder. In the *International Statistical Classification of Diseases and Related Health Problems* (ICD-10) the disorder requires a history of at least six unexplained symptoms from at least two of the following symptom groups: gastrointestinal, cardio-

TABLE 2.1. DSM-IV Diagnostic Criteria for Somatization Disorder

A. A history of many physical complaints beginning before age 30 years that occur over a period of several years and result in treatment being sought or significant impairment in social, occupational, or other important areas of functioning.

B. Each of the following criteria must have been met, with individual symptoms occurring at any time during the course of the disturbance.
    (1) *four pain symptoms*: a history of pain related to at least four different sites or functions (e.g., head, abdomen, back, joints, extremities, chest, rectum, during menstruation, during sexual intercourse, or during urination)
    (2) *two gastrointestinal symptoms*: a history of at least two gastrointestinal symptoms other than pain (e.g., nausea, bloating, vomiting other than during pregnancy, diarrhea, or intolerance of several different foods)
    (3) *one sexual symptom*: a history of at least one sexual or reproductive symptom other than pain (e.g., sexual indifference, erectile or ejaculatory dysfunction, irregular menses, excessive menstrual bleeding, vomiting throughout pregnancy)
    (4) *one pseudoneurological symptom*: a history of at least one symptom or deficit suggesting a neurological condition not limited to pain (conversion symptoms such as impaired coordination or balance, paralysis or localized weakness, difficulty swallowing or lump in throat, aphonia, urinary retention, hallucinations, loss of touch or pain sensation, double vision, blindness, deafness, seizures; dissociative symptoms such as amnesia; or loss of consciousness other than fainting)

C. Either (1) or (2):
    (1) after appropriate investigation, each of the symptoms in Criterion B cannot be fully explained by a known general medical condition or the direct effects of a substance (e.g., a drug of abuse, a medication)
    (2) when there is a related general medical condition, the physical complaints or resulting social or occupational impairment are in excess of what would be expected from the history, physical examination, or laboratory findings

D. The symptoms are not intentionally produced or feigned (as in Factitious Disorder or Malingering).

Note. From American Psychiatric Association (1994). Copyright 1994 by the American Psychiatric Association. Reprinted by permission.

vascular, genitourinary, and skin/pain (World Health Organization, 1993). In all three versions of DSM and in ICD-10, symptoms counted toward the diagnosis of somatization disorder must be either medically unexplained or experienced in excess of what would be expected from physical examination and laboratory findings. In addition, ICD-10 requires that each symptom be distressing enough to prompt the repeated seeking of medical treatment. In DSM-III and its later revisions, unexplained physical symptoms counted toward the somatization disorder diagnosis must have either prompted the seeking of medical treatment or impaired the individual's functioning.

Not only do the various versions of DSM and ICD establish different symptom thresholds for the diagnosis of somatization disorder, but they also utilize different lists of criterial symptoms. The symptom lists for somatization disorder according to DSM-III, DSM-III-R, DSM-IV, and ICD-10, as well as the lists used for hysteria (Feighner et al., 1972; Guze, 1967; Perley & Guze, 1962) are displayed in Table 2.2. The 59-item Perley–Guze/Feighner list was shortened for DSM-III largely by eliminating its psychological symptoms (e.g., nervousness, depressed feelings). Additional, though minimal, reductions to the original list were made for DSM-III-R, and it was condensed further for DSM-IV. DSM-III and DSM-III-R fashion a purely somatic variety of hysteria, while DSM-IV includes hallucinations, one of the original psychological symptoms from Perley and Guze's list. This symptom is not associated with somatization disorder in either DSM-III or DSM-III-R. ICD-10 somatization disorder bears little resemblance to Perley and Guze's hysteria. Symptoms listed in ICD-10 are significantly fewer in number, including none of the menstrual or pseudoneurological symptoms considered the cardinal features of the original syndrome (Guze & Perley, 1963). In ICD-10 a distinction is drawn between somatization/somatoform disorders and dissociative/conversion disorders. Pseudoneurological symptoms fall into the latter category according to the WHO.

A decade since the publication of the most recent classification systems (ICD-10 and DSM-IV), discord continues over appropriate symptom lists and symptom thresholds for diagnosing somatization disorder. All four versions of somatization disorder are predictive of important clinical outcomes, such as overuse of medical services and functional impairment (Bass & Murphy, 1991; Gureje, Simon, et al., 1997; Smith et al., 1986a; Swartz, Blazer, George, & Landerman, 1986). There is little evidence, however, supporting DSM-IV's and ICD-10's subgrouping of symptoms (Liu, Clark, & Eaton, 1997). Also, given the greater likelihood that women will experience and report somatization symptoms than will men, some investigators have encouraged the continued use of different symptom thresholds for men and women, as in DSM-III (Liu et al., 1997). And, although most research suggests that the criteria from the various versions of DSM somatization disorder (and from Perley and Guze's hysteria) identify roughly identical groups of patients, ICD-10's criteria for somatization disorder may indeed designate a different group of patients (Rief et al., 1996; Yutzy et al., 1995).

TABLE 2.2. Symptom Lists for Classification Systems of Somatization Disorder/Hysteria

Perley–Guze/Feighner	DSM-III	DSM-III-R	DSM-IV	ICD-10
		Pseudoneurological symptoms		
Paralysis	Paralysis or muscle weakness	Paralysis or muscle weakness	Paralysis or localized weakness[b]	
Trouble walking (ataxia)[a]	Trouble walking	Trouble walking	Impaired coordination or balance[b]	
Lump in throat	Difficulty swallowing	Difficulty swallowing	Difficulty swallowing or lump in throat[b]	
Aphonia	Loss of voice	Loss of voice	Aphonia[b]	
Deafness	Deafness	Deafness	Deafness[b]	
	Double vision	Double vision	Double vision[b]	
Blindness	Blindness	Blindness	Blindness[b]	
Fits or convulsions	Seizures or convulsions	Seizure or convulsion	Seizures[b]	
Urinary retention	Urinary retention or difficulty urinating	Urinary retention or difficulty urinating	Urinary retention[b]	
Fainting spells	Fainting or loss of consciousness	Fainting or loss of consciousness	Loss of consciousness (other than fainting)[b]	
Amnesia	Memory loss	Amnesia	Amnesia[b]	
Visual blurring	Blurred vision	Blurred vision		
Anesthesia			Loss of touch or pain sensation[b]	Unpleasant numbness or tingling[c]
Hallucinations			Hallucinations[b]	
Unconsciousness				
Weakness				
Other conversion symptoms[a]				

Gastrointestinal symptoms

Nausea	Nausea	Nausea (other than motion sickness)	Nausea[e]	Bad taste in mouth or coated tongue[d]
				Nausea[d]
Vomiting	Vomiting (other than during pregnancy)	Vomiting (other than during pregnancy)	Vomiting (other than during pregnancy)[e]	Vomiting or regurgitation[d]
Abdominal bloating	Bloating (gassy)	Bloating (gassy)	Bloating[e]	Feeling bloated or full of gas[d]
Diarrhea	Diarrhea	Diarrhea	Diarrhea[e]	Frequent and loose bowels or anal discharge[d]
Food intolerances	Food intolerance	Food intolerance	Food intolerance[e]	
Constipation				
Anorexia				
Weight loss				
Marked fluctuations in weight				

Sexual/menstrual symptoms

Menstrual irregularity	Menstrual irregularity	Irregular menstrual periods	Irregular menses[f]	
Excessive menstrual bleeding	Excessive menstrual bleeding	Excessive menstrual bleeding	Excessive menstrual bleeding[f]	
Amenorrhea				
Vomiting throughout pregnancy	Severe vomiting throughout pregnancy	Vomiting throughout pregnancy	Vomiting throughout pregnancy[f]	
Sexual indifference	Sexual indifference	Sexual indifference	Sexual indifference[f]	
Sexual frigidity		Impotence	Erectile or ejaculatory dysfunction[f]	
Other sexual difficulties	Lack of pleasure during intercourse			Unusual or copious vaginal discharge[i]

(continued)

TABLE 2.2. (continued)

Perley–Guze/Feighner	DSM-III	DSM-III-R	DSM-IV	ICD-10
		Pain symptoms		
Abdominal pain	Abdominal pain	Abdominal pain (other than when menstruating)	Pain in abdomen[g]	Abdominal pain[d]
Back pain	Pain in back	Back pain	Pain in back[g]	
Joint pain	Pain in joints	Joint pain	Pain in joints[g]	Pain in limbs, extremities, or joints[c]
Extremity pain	Pain in extremities	Pain in extremities	Pain in extremities[g]	
Burning in sexual organs, mouth, or rectum	Pain in genital area (other than during sex)	Burning in sexual organs or rectum (other than during sex)	Pain in rectum[g]	Unpleasant genital sensations[i]
Pain during urination	Pain on urination	Pain during urination	Pain during urination[g]	Dysuria or frequent urination[i]
Dysmenorrhea	Painful menstruation	Painful menstruation	Pain during menstruation[g]	
Dyspareunia	Pain during intercourse	Pain during intercourse	Pain during intercourse[g]	
Other bodily pain	Other pain (other than headaches)	Other pain (other than headache)		
Headache	Headache		Pain in head[g]	
		Cardiovascular symptoms		
Chest pain	Chest pain	Chest pain	Pain in chest[g]	Chest pains[h]
Breathing difficulty	Shortness of breath	Shortness of breath when not exerting oneself		Breathlessness without exertion[h]
Palpitation	Palpitations	Palpitations		
Dizziness	Dizziness	Dizziness		

20

Feeling sickly most of life	Feeling sickly much of life	Other symptoms
Fatigue		Blotchiness or discoloration of skin[c]
Anxiety attacks		
Nervousness		
Fears		
Depressed feelings		
Quitting work or other functional limitations because feeling sick		
Crying easily		
Feeling life is hopeless		
Thinking a good deal about dying		
Wanting to die		
Thinking of suicide		
Suicide attempts		

[a]Included in Feighner criteria only (i.e., not in Perley & Guze's [1962] original symptom list).
[b]Categorized in the pseudoneurological cluster of symptoms in DSM-IV.
[c]Categorized in the skin/pain cluster of symptoms in ICD-10.
[d]Categorized in the gastrointestinal cluster of symptoms in ICD-10.
[e]Categorized in the gastrointestinal cluster of symptoms in DSM-IV.
[f]Categorized in the sexual/menstrual cluster of symptoms in DSM-IV.
[g]Categorized in the pain cluster of symptoms in DSM-IV.
[h]Categorized in the cardiovascular cluster of symptoms in ICD-10.
[i]Categorized in the genitourinary cluster of symptoms in ICD-10.

Despite the differences among the specific criteria for somatization disorder, the essence of somatization disorder according to any classification system is *chronic* unexplained physical symptoms. According to the diagnostic criteria described in DSM-III, DSM-III-R, and DSM-IV, at least some of the somatization symptoms must have occurred prior to the patient's 30th birthday (American Psychiatric Association, 1980, 1987, 1994). The ICD-10 criteria require the patient to report experiencing somatization symptoms for at least 2 years but do not specify at what age the symptoms must have first occurred (World Health Organization, 1993). The course of somatization disorder tends to be characterized by symptoms that wax and wane, remitting only to return later and/or be replaced by new unexplained physical symptoms (Lieb et al., 2002). Thus, an important feature of somatization disorder is that it is a polysymptomatic disorder whose requisite symptoms need not be manifested concurrently.

This persistent, polysymptomatic disorder is difficult to identify in clinical practice. Spotting it requires the clinician to review patients' past and current symptomatology and to determine whether each physical complaint is medically unexplained or whether it produces discomfort in excess of that expected from the organic pathology observed. Furthermore, the clinician must establish whether the symptom has brought about functional impairment, the use of medication, and/or the seeking of medical treatment. Time limitations may prevent clinicians from investigating so many symptoms that may have occurred over so long an interval. For example, a patient who has a history of multiple unexplained physical symptoms but is presently experiencing only unexplained and debilitating back pain may not receive a diagnosis of somatization disorder if the clinician asks only about the patient's current symptomatology. Also, clinicians may hesitate to make the somatization diagnosis because of uncertainty regarding potential underlying organic pathology. Because of these complex requirements for a somatization disorder diagnosis, it is likely underdiagnosed in medical and psychiatric clinics (Fabrega, Mezzich, Jacob, & Ulrich, 1988; Fink, Sorensen, Engberg, Holm, & Munk-Jorgensen, 1999; Peveler, Kilkenny, & Kinmonth, 1997).

The differences in the diagnostic criteria of DSM-III, DSM-III-R, DSM-IV, and ICD-10, though subtle in some instances, may be responsible for some of the inconsistencies in the epidemiological findings that are described below. Some epidemiological research has suggested that somatization disorder is relatively rare. In the Epidemiologic Catchment Area (ECA) study, the largest survey of somatization disorder (carried out in a *community* sample of 20,000 people across five sites in the United States), the lifetime prevalence of DSM-III somatization disorder was 0.13% (Robins & Reiger, 1991). Prior research had resulted in higher estimates for Perley and Guze's hysteria, ranging from 0.4 to 2% of the population (Weissman, Myers, & Harding, 1978; Woodruff, Clayton, & Guze, 1971). Not surprisingly, somatization disorder appears to be more common in primary care settings than in community populations. In the WHO Cross-National Study of Mental Disorders in Primary Care, in which 5,438 *primary care* patients at 15 centers in 14 countries were assessed, the prevalence of somatization disorder was 0.9% and 2.8%, as defined by DSM-III-R and ICD-10, respectively (Gureje, Simon, et al., 1997). Smaller studies conducted in primary care settings have estimated the prevalence of DSM-III-R somatization disorder to range from 1% in a sample of 685 patients (Kirmayer & Robbins, 1991) to 5% of a sample of 222 patients (Peveler et al., 1997).

For a number of reasons, several authorities suggest the actual prevalence of somatization disorder may be substantially higher than the literature suggests. First, autobiographical memory of past psychiatric symptoms, including somatization symptoms, is unreliable. Individuals seem to forget (or at least fail to report) previously reported symptoms that are no longer troublesome (Simon & Gureje, 1999; Simon & Von Korff, 1995). Given that the somatization disorder diagnosis requires patients to describe both current and remitted symptoms, the latter often not recalled, the true occurrence of somatization disorder is probably underestimated in these studies. Second, the diagnosis of somatization disorder necessitates that a physical examination and diagnostic tests be performed, or that medical records be reviewed, to determine the nature of each symptom. Such extensive investigations of physical symptoms are too costly to incorporate into large epidemiological studies. The third argument for the underestimation of prevalence rates has to do with the conjecture that physicians are more likely to make the somatization diagnosis than are nonphysician diagnosticians (Martin, 1991; Swartz, Blazer, et al., 1986). Presumably, physicians are better able to distinguish between a medically sound explanation for a symptom and the patient's medical-sounding explanation for that symptom. Because nonphysicians conducted assessments without access to medical records in the ECA and WHO studies cited above, somatization disorder may have been underdiagnosed in those studies. At the one site in the ECA study where physicians evaluated symptom reports to determine whether symptoms were medically explained, the prevalence of somatization disorder was higher than at the other sites (Swartz, Blazer, et al., 1986).

Subthreshold Somatization

Some investigators have encouraged a broadening of the somatization construct to include the many patients affected by unexplained symptoms not numerous enough to meet criteria for full somatization disorder. Both ICD-10 and DSM-IV include residual diagnostic categories for subthreshold somatization cases. In DSM-IV (American Psychiatric Association, 1994), "undifferentiated somatoform disorder" is a diagnosis characterized by one or more medically unexplained physical symptoms lasting for at least 6 months (see Table 2.3). ICD-10's undifferentiated somatoform disorder category differs from DSM-IV's in that ICD-10 requires multiple unexplained symptoms lasting for at least 6 months (World Health Organization, 1993). ICD-10 provides an additional category for subthreshold somatization disorder, "somatoform autonomic dysfunction," for cases of three or more unexplained symptoms of autonomic arousal (World Health Organization, 1993). We are aware of no published data that establish the validity of any of these three diagnostic categories.

Two research teams have suggested categories for subthreshold somatization other than those described in DSM-IV and ICD-10. Escobar,

---

TABLE 2.3. DSM-IV Diagnostic Criteria for Undifferentiated Somatoform Disorder

A. One or more physical complaints (e.g., fatigue, loss of appetite, gastrointestinal or urinary complaints).

B. Either (1) or (2):
   (1) after appropriate investigation, the symptoms cannot be fully explained by a known general medical condition or the direct effects of a substance (e.g., a drug of abuse, a medication)
   (2) when there is a related general medical condition, the physical complaints or resulting social or occupational impairment are in excess of what would be expected from the history, physical examination, or laboratory findings

C. The symptoms cause clinically significant distress or impairment in social, occupational, or other important areas of functioning.

D. The duration of the disturbance is at least 6 months.

E. The disturbance is not better accounted for by another mental disorder (e.g., another Somatoform Disorder, Sexual Dysfunction, Mood Disorder, Anxiety Disorder, Sleep Disorder, or Psychotic Disorder).

F. The symptom is not intentionally produced or feigned (as in Factitious Disorder or Malingering).

Note. From American Psychiatric Association (1994). Copyright 1994 by the American Psychiatric Association. Reprinted by permission.

Burnam, Karno, Forsythe, and Golding (1987) proposed the label "abridged somatization" to be applied to men experiencing four or more unexplained physical symptoms or to women experiencing six or more unexplained physical symptoms. Kroenke and colleagues (1997) suggested the category of "multisomatoform disorder" to describe men or women currently experiencing at least three unexplained physical symptoms and reporting a 2-year history of somatization. Both of these subthreshold somatization categories appear to be significantly more prevalent than is full somatization disorder, described earlier. Abridged somatization has been observed in 4.4% of community samples (Escobar, Burnam, et al., 1987) and 16.6–22% of primary care samples (Escobar, Waitzkin, Silver, Gara, & Holman, 1998; Gureje, Simon, et al., 1997; Kirmayer & Robbins, 1991). The occurrence of multisomatoform disorder has been estimated at 8.2% of primary care patients (Kroenke et al., 1997).

The demographic characteristic most often associated with somatization is sex. In the ECA study, women were 10 times more likely to meet criteria for somatization disorder than were men (Swartz, Landermann, George, Blazer, & Escobar, 1991). Sex differences, though not as extreme, also have been found in most studies employing subthreshold somatization categories, such as Escobar's abridged somatization or Kroenke's multisomatoform disorder (Escobar, Rubio-Stipec, Canino, & Karno, 1989; Kroenke et al., 1997). A more complex picture of the association between sex and somatization was suggested by the WHO's Cross-National study in which female primary care patients were more likely to meet ICD-10 criteria for full somatization disorder, but no more likely to meet Escobar's abridged somatization criteria, than were their male counterparts (Gureje, Simon, et al., 1997). At least on the severe end of the continuum, somatization disorder is uncommon in men. Sex differences are less obvious in the various subthreshold syndromes.

Current thinking is that the low prevalence of somatization disorder in men may be explained, in part, by stereotypical male traits, such as a disinclination to admit discomfort and an unwillingness to seek medical treatment (see Wool & Barsky, 1994, for review). Also physicians may be less likely to consider somatization as a possible explanation for a man's symptoms than for a woman's symptoms (Golding, Smith, & Kashner, 1991). Gender biases may cause physicians to communicate with and treat male patients differently from the ways in which they communicate with and treat female patients. At this juncture, we have only conjectural explanations for the different rates of somatization in men and women.

Ethnicity, race, and education have also been associated with somatization disorder and subthreshold somatization. Epidemiological research has shown patients with somatization were more likely to be female, nonwhite, and less educated than nonsomatizers (Gureje, Simon, et al., 1997; Robins & Reiger, 1991). Findings on ethnicity have been less consistent across studies. In the ECA study, Hispanics were no more likely to meet criteria for somatization disorder than were non-Hispanics (Robins & Reiger, 1991). The WHO study, conducted in 14 different countries, revealed a higher incidence of somatization, as defined by either ICD-10 or Escobar's abridged criteria, in Latin American countries than in the United States (Gureje, Simon, et al., 1997).

Findings on the relationship between age and somatization have been somewhat consistent. Most studies indicate that somatization disorder and abridged somatization are more common in middle-aged and older patients (over 45 years of age) than in younger patients (Gureje, Simon, et al., 1997; Swartz, Blazer, et al., 1986). Some research, however, has detected no association between somatization disorder and age (Robins & Reiger, 1991). Children and adolescents, of course, are extremely unlikely to meet criteria for somatization disorder (and cannot, if one uses DSM-IV criteria), perhaps because they have not lived long enough to acquire enough clinically significant somatization symptoms, especially sexual and menstrual symptoms.

Functional Somatic Syndromes

The term "functional somatic syndrome" is used to describe groups of co-occurring symptoms that are medically unexplained. Polysymptomatic functional somatic syndromes frequently encountered by both mental health and primary care practitioners include irritable bowel syndrome (IBS), chronic fatigue syndrome (CFS), and fibromyalgia.

CFS is characterized by unexplained fatigue, lasting at least 6 months, that causes substantial reduction in activities. At least four of the following symptoms must have co-occurred with the fatigue: significant memory impairment or concentration difficulties, sore throat, tender lymph nodes, muscle pain, joint pain, headache, nonrestorative sleep, and postexertional fatigue (Fukuda et al., 1994). CFS's prevalence has been estimated to be 0.002–0.6% in the general population and 2.6% in primary care settings (Jason et al., 1999; Reyes et al., 2003; Wessely, Chadler, Hirsch, Wallace, & Wright, 1997). Women are more likely than men to suffer from CFS (Jason et al., 1999; Reyes et al., 2003). Although the incidence of CFS appears to be elevated in minority groups (especially Hispanics and African Americans), larger epidemiological studies are required to confirm these findings (Jason et al., 1999).

A diagnosis of fibromyalgia is given for chronic widespread pain and multiple tender points that have no known biological basis and are accompanied by nonrestorative sleep, fatigue, and malaise (Wolfe et al., 1990). Fibromyalgia has been estimated to occur in about 2% of the U.S. population and in 6–20% of general medical outpatients (Wolfe, Ross, Anderson, Russell, & Hebert, 1995). Like the other functional somatic syndromes, fibromyalgia is more likely to affect women than men (Wolfe et al., 1995).

IBS is characterized by persistent abdominal pain along with altered bowel habits and abdominal distension that cannot be explained by organic pathology (Thompson, Dotevall, Drossman, Heaton, & Kruis, 1989). It has been estimated that 8–20% of the U.S. population, 12% of primary care patients (Drossman, Whitehead, & Camilleri, 1997), and 22–28% of gastroenterologists' patients are afflicted with IBS (Harvey, Salih, & Read, 1983; Thompson & Heaton, 1980). The ratio of female to male patients diagnosed with IBS has been estimated to be 2:1 (Drossman et al., 1993).

Our decision to aggregate the research on somatization disorder, subthreshold somatization, CFS, fibromyalgia, and IBS may invite controversy. Some medical specialists, focusing on the bodily organ or somatic system of their specialization, assume these disorders have distinct pathophysiological causes and draw sharp distinctions among these syndromes. Other authorities suggest these syndromes should be viewed as one disorder. After all, many patients diagnosed with one functional somatic syndrome meet diagnostic criteria for one or more of the other functional somatic syndromes, resulting in multi-system comorbid functional syndromes (Buchwald & Garrity, 1994; Goldenberg, Simms, Geiger, & Komaroff, 1990; Veale, Kavanagh, Fielding, & Fitzgerald, 1991; Yunus, Masi, & Aldag, 1989a). Also, investigators have noted similarities in the illness behaviors, illness beliefs, and psychological functioning of patients diagnosed with one of these somatization syndromes (Barsky & Borus, 1999; Rief, Hiller, & Margraf, 1998; Wessely, Nimnuan, & Sharpe, 1999). As will be discussed later in this chapter and in Chapter 3, patients with somatization tend to adopt a sick role (Parsons, 1951), overutilizing medical services and withdrawing from their normal activities. They tend to assume their symptoms are signs of a serious, disabling illness that is likely to worsen; they think catastrophically about their health. They frequently suffer from concurrent emotional disorders. Because we have concluded that the research suggests greater similarity than distinction among the various categories of somatization, we have adopted the convention of using the terms "somatization" and "somatization syndromes" to refer to and encompass the all the poly-symptomatic syndromes, including CFS, fibromyalgia, IBS, abridged somatization, multisomatoform disorder, and somatization disorder.

Differential Diagnosis

Within the context of DSM's dualistic framework that distinguishes between mental disorders and general medical conditions, somatization symptoms cannot be accounted for entirely by the latter. Before the diagnosis of somatization can be made, potential underlying medical conditions must be excluded. Medical conditions that are most likely to account for the multisystem complaints associated with full somatization disorder include multiple sclerosis, hyperparathyroidism, and systemic lupus erythematosus. Countless other medical illnesses could account for single-system or single-symptom complaints, and there are numerous "borderline" symptoms for which morphological anomalies can be measured but fail to correspond to subjective distress (e.g., disc herniation and its relation to back pain). Thus, a close collaboration with patients' medical practitioners is required to recognize and treat organic pathology.

This is not to say that somatization and organic illness cannot co-occur. Many patients with medically explained symptoms also experience somatization symptoms (Chaturvedi, Maguire, & Somashekar, 2006; Heckman et al., 2002; Sonino et al., 2004). These cases, in fact, may be the most difficult to treat (Dickinson et al., 2003). For example, in patients with cancer, comorbid somatization symptoms have been shown to complicate diagnosis, treatment, and cancer outcome (Chaturvedi et al., 2006). General medical conditions also may be the original causes of symptoms that are judged to be excessive or disproportionate in relation to the organic cause and, therefore, part of a pattern of somatization.

A second area of distinction is between somatization and hypochondriasis. Hypochondriasis is defined in DSM-IV as a preoccupation with fears that or the belief that one has a serious, undiagnosed disease (American Psychiatric Association, 1994). To meet full criteria for hypochondriasis, the preoccupation must persist for at least six months despite medical assurance of no organic illness (American Psychiatric Association, 1994). Although most patients with hypochondriasis experience somatic symptoms, it is not the somatic symptoms themselves that impair functioning in hypochondriasis. Instead, in hypochondriasis, it is the fears about the meaning of the physical symptoms that cause distress, dysfunction, and overuse of healthcare services. Whether hypochondriasis is more accurately represented by a discrete diagnosis or by a dimension is a subject of debate (Creed & Barsky, 2004). Not only DSM-IV defined hypochondriasis, but excessive health anxiety that does not meet all of DSM-IV's criteria for a diagnosis of hypochondriasis is associated with significant impairment and cost (Gureje, Ustun, & Simon, 1997; Looper & Kirmayer, 2001).

While the boundaries between DSM-IV somatization disorder and hypochondriasis can be distinguished, there remains significant overlap between these constructs. The co-occurrence of DSM-IV somatization disorder and DSM-IV hypochondriasis is infrequent (Barsky, Wyshak, & Klerman, 1992; Escobar, Gara, et al., 1998). Only about 20% of patients with hypochondriasis meet DSM criteria for somatization disorder, and about 20% of patients with somatization disorder meet DSM criteria for hypochondriasis (Barsky et al., 1992; Escobar, Gara, et al., 1998). Nevertheless, many patients with somatization have hypochondriacal beliefs, and many patients with hypochondriasis experience somatization symptoms (Creed & Barsky, 2004). As will be discussed below, similar treatments have been shown to be effective for somatization and hypochondriasis.

The presentation of an anxiety disorder may resemble that of somatization (Smith et al., 2005). Patients experiencing panic attacks report multiple medically unexplained physical symptoms. The difference between somatization and panic disorder is that the symptoms of the latter occur with a sudden and acute onset, whereas the former are more insidious (American Psychiatric Association, 1994). Likewise, generalized anxiety disorder may present itself as a largely somatic set of complaints, including muscle tension and pain, fatigue, and insomnia. The distinguishing feature of generalized anxiety disorder is the pervasive worry that accompanies the somatic symptoms (American Psychiatric Association, 1994). Although somatic symptoms occurring during a panic attack or in the context of generalized anxiety disorder are not counted toward the diagnosis of somatization, there are many patients who report comorbid somatization and panic disorder or generalized anxiety disorder (Brown, Golding, & Smith, 1990; Fink, 1995; Katon, Von Korff, & Lin, 1992; Robins & Reiger, 1991).

So, too, patients experiencing depression may present somatic symptoms rather than a dysphoric mood or anhedonia to healthcare professionals (Smith et al., 2005). Somatic presentations of depression often involve symptoms such as fatigue, weakness, gastrointestinal distress, headaches, other pain symptoms, or hypochondriacal beliefs (Lipowski, 1988), symptoms common in somatoform disorders. Upon questioning, however, patients with depression acknowledge diminished mood or interest (American Psychiatric Association, 1994), and the course of their somatic symptoms tends to mirror that of their mood symptoms (Lipowski, 1988). On the other hand, the course of somatic symptoms associated with somatization may not be tied as closely to mood.

The overlap between somatization and depression is high. When depression and somatization are conceived and measured as dimensions, they are positively correlated (Katon et al., 1991; Simon et al., 1999). When defined by DSM categories, up to 50% of patients with somatization disorder meet criteria for a lifetime diagnosis of major depressive disorder (Simon & Von Korff, 1991). Relatively few patients meeting criteria for major depressive disorder meet criteria for somatization disorder, though up to 75% of patients with depression report at least one medically unexplained symptom (Corruble & Guelfi, 2000; Simon et al., 1999).

Additional evidence for the overlap among somatization, anxiety, and depressive disorders comes from two other areas of research: longitudinal research on somatization syndromes and research on the family members of patients with somatization. Longitudinal research not only suggests somatization syndromes are relatively stable, though with some shifts in symptomatic focus (Lieb et al., 2002), but also may be predictive of future depression and/or anxiety disorders (Hotopf, Carr, Mayou, Wadsworth, & Wesseley, 1998; Zwaigenbaum, Szatmari, Boyle, & Offord, 1999). A preexisting depression or anxiety disorder is associated with a future somatization syndrome (Gureje & Simon, 1999). Family members of patients with somatization appear to have higher-than-expected rates of depression and anxiety disorders (Hudson, Arnold, Keck, Auchenbach, & Pope, 2004).

CLINICAL CHARACTERISTICS

Much attention has focused on the illness behavior of patients with somatization and the resulting impact of that behavior on the healthcare system. These patients disproportionately use and misuse healthcare services. When standard diagnostic evaluations fail to uncover organic pathology, patients with somatization tend to seek additional medical procedures, often from several different physicians. Patients may even subject themselves to unnecessary hospitalizations and surgeries, which introduce the risk of iatrogenic illness (Fink, 1992). One study found that patients diagnosed with DSM-III somatization disorder incurred nine times the U.S. per capita healthcare cost (Smith et al.,

1986a). Abridged somatization, multisomatoform disorder, CFS, fibromyalgia, and IBS all have been associated with high healthcare utilization (Barsky, Orav, & Bates, 2005; Bombardier & Buchwald, 1996; Kroenke et al., 1997; Leong et al., 2003; Lloyd & Pender, 1992; Restak et al., 2003). Pilowsky (1969) used the phrase "abnormal illness behavior" to describe the dysfunctional behaviors in which patients with hypochondriasis and somatization engage. According to Pilowsky, inappropriate healthcare-seeking behavior is motivated by fear of disease and/or the potential rewards of the "sick role." This is not to say that all somatizers are overutilizers of mainstream medical services. Some focus entirely on complementary and alternative healthcare, and some cease to seek any remedy after a lengthy history of unsuccessful treatment.

The abnormal illness behavior of patients with somatization extends beyond medical offices and hospitals to patients' workplaces and households. Somatizers withdraw from both productive and pleasurable activities because of discomfort, fatigue, and/or fears of exacerbating their symptoms. Investigators have found 18–60% of patients diagnosed with somatization disorder to be receiving disability payments from either their employers or the government (Allen, Woolfolk, Escobar, Gara, & Hamer, 2006; Bass & Murphy, 1991). Estimates of unemployment among patients with somatization disorder range from 36% to 83% (Allen et al., 2006; Smith et al., 1986a; Yutzy et al., 1995). Whether working outside their homes or not, these patients report substantial functional impairment. Some investigators have found that patients with somatization disorder are bedridden for 2–7 days per month (Katon et al., 1991; Smith et al., 1986a). Likewise, patients diagnosed with subsyndrome somatization or a functional somatic syndrome report significant reductions in their productive activities (Allen, Gara, Escobar, Waitzkin, & Cohen-Silver, 2001; Bombardier & Buchwald, 1996; Drossman et al., 1993; Escobar, Golding, et al., 1987; Gureje, Simon, et al., 1997; Kroenke et al., 1997; Leong et al., 2003; Wolfe et al., 1997). In fact, Katon and colleagues (1991) found a linear relationship between the number of unexplained symptoms and the severity of functional impairment.

In addition to their physical complaints, most patients with somatization complain of psychiatric distress. As many as 80% of patients meeting criteria for somatization disorder, CFS, fibromyalgia, or IBS meet criteria for another lifetime DSM Axis I disorder, usually an anxiety or mood disorder (Bass & Murphy, 1991; Clark et al., 1995; Epstein et al., 1999; Ford, Miller, Eastwood, & Eastwood, 1987; Swartz, Blazer, et al., 1986). When investigators consider only current psychiatric diagnoses, rates of psychiatric comorbidity associated with somatization syndromes are closer to 50% (Allen et al., 2006; Camilleri & Choi, 1997; Epstein et al., 1999; Simon & Von Korff, 1991). Also, overall severity of psychological distress, defined as the number of psychological symptoms reported, correlates positively with the number of functional somatic symptoms reported (Katon et al., 1991; Simon & Von Korff, 1991).

Although the association between physical and psychological symptoms has been clearly established, the mechanism explaining this association has yet to be identified. Mechanisms that may be involved in this relationship include the following:

1. A common physiological, cognitive, or personality disturbance may underlie both functional somatic and psychological symptoms.
2. Mood disturbances may increase the likelihood of somatic complaints by lowering pain thresholds and triggering symptom amplification.
3. Chronic, unresolved, disabling physical discomfort may create emotional distress.

Whatever the mechanism might be, the frequent co-occurrence of psychological and somatization symptoms seems to be inconsistent with the psychodynamic conceptualization of somatoform conversion as a defense against negative affect.

Only a few personality types and cognitive styles have consistently been ascribed to patients with somatization. Patients with somatization disorder, CFS, fibromyalgia, and IBS all tend to score higher than medical patients and/or nonpatient controls on scales of neuroticism and negative affect (Blakely et al., 1991; Epstein et al., 1999; Noyes et al., 2001; Talley, Boyce, & Jones, 1998). Also, somatoform patients tend to amplify their somatic sensations and express catastrophic beliefs and helpless feelings about their symptoms (Barsky, 1992; Burckhardt & Bjelle, 1996; Nicassio, Schuman, Radojevic, & Weisman, 1999; Rief, Hiller, & Margraf, 1998). Thus, there is a hyperreactivity to both emotional and physical stimuli that may exaggerate their expected effects.

Another characteristic often thought to be associated with somatization is a history of abuse or of trauma. Women who have been physically or sexually assaulted during childhood or adulthood are more likely to report multiple, medically unexplained physical symptoms than are women who report no history of abuse (McCauley et al., 1997). A self-report of trauma is more common in women diagnosed with functional somatic syndromes, such as fibromyalgia or IBS, than in women diagnosed with organic diseases, such as rheumatoid arthritis (Walker et al., 1997) or inflammatory bowel disease (Walker, Gelfand, Gelfand, & Katon, 1995). Similarly, women with chronic pelvic pain report more childhood sexual and physical abuse than do nonpain gynecology patients (Harrop-Griffiths et al., 1988). Yet, studies examining the relationship between somatization and reported abuse have not yielded a consistent pattern of results. Some investigators have found no association between abuse history and somatization (Hobbis, Turpin, & Read, 2002; Taylor & Leonard, 2001). The only study in which victims of childhood abuse were followed *prospectively* into adulthood failed to show a link between childhood victimization and functional somatic symptoms (Raphael, Widom, & Lange, 2001). Notably, *retrospective* self-reports from Raphael and colleagues' adult sample did show an association between abuse history and somatization symptoms. More recent research has found an association between somatization and negative family environments (e.g., cold, critical parents) but no specific association between somatization and childhood abuse (Brown, Schrag, & Trimble, 2005; Lackner, Gudleski, & Blanchard, 2004). In summary, the strength of the association between somatization and abuse is unclear. Methodological factors, such as using retrospective self-reports of abuse versus following patients prospectively, may account for the discrepancy in findings. Another methodological variation in the above-cited studies is the population from which study participants were selected (i.e., medical patients versus community members). It may be that patients with somatization who seek medical treatment for their unexplained physical symptoms are more likely to report abuse histories than are those not seeking treatment (Aaron et al., 1997; Drossman et al., 1990).

The clinical profile of a hypersensitive patient who meets DSM criteria for an anxiety or depressive disorder and labels herself a victim of trauma may evoke the image of a typical psychiatric patient. In fact, many patients with somatization willingly seek mental health services for their depressed and/or anxious moods (Zoccolillo & Cloninger, 1986); however, they rarely seek psychiatric treatment for somatization symptoms per se (Smith et al., 1986a). For patients with somatization, physical symptoms are interpreted as signs of a somatic illness that require standard, somatic medical treatment. These patients may choose not to discuss their "medical" complaints with their mental health practitioners. Providers of mental health services may be ill-equipped to rule out organic pathology and therefore choose to avoid discussions of somatic symptoms and/or encourage the seeking of standard medical care for them and, in so doing, unwittingly promote patients' dysfunctional illness behavior. Whatever benefits patients with somatization derive from psychiatric treatment seem not to extend to their unexplained physical symptoms.

TREATMENT OUTCOME RESEARCH
Pharmacological Interventions

Many investigators have examined the impact of pharmacological treatments on somatization syndromes, most often on one of the functional somatic syndromes. Despite the sizeable body of research on pharmacological treatments for functional somatic syndromes and the frequency with which these syndromes are treated with medication, few medications appear to provide "clinically meaningful" relief. What follows is a brief summary of the controlled medication trials that have been conducted with somatization patients. Detailed reviews of this literature can be found elsewhere (Arnold, Keck, & Welge, 2000; Jailwala, Imperiale, & Kroenke, 2000; Klein, 1988; Whiting et al., 2001).

Although not one controlled trial has been conducted on the efficacy of a pharmacological agent for full somatization disorder, the efficacy of specific medications on subthreshold somatization has been examined in four randomized controlled studies. Three studies were conducted in Germany and included patients meeting ICD-10 criteria for somatization disorder, undifferentiated somatoform disorder, or somatoform autonomic dysfunction. In the first study, treatment with opipramol, a tricyclic compound, reduced somatic symptoms more than did treatment with placebo (Volz, Moller, Reimann, & Stoll, 2000). In the second and third studies, patients treated with St. John's wort, Hypericum perforatum, experienced greater improvement in somatic symptoms than did patients treated with placebo (Muller, Mannel, Murck, & Rahlfs, 2004; Volz, Murck, Kasper, & Moller, 2002). The most recent study suggested venlafaxine is a more effective pain reliever than is placebo in depressed and anxious primary care patients who meet criteria for multisomatoform disorder (Kroenke, Messina, Benattia, Graepel, & Musgnung, 2006). Although opipramol, St. John's wort, and venlafaxine outperformed placebo, none of these studies provides evidence that a majority of participants experienced either "clinically meaningful" or lasting relief from these agents.

Antidepressant treatment for functional somatic syndromes has received some support in controlled trials. On the whole, CFS patients have not benefited from antidepressant medication (Whiting et al., 2001). The evidence for the efficacy of antidepressants for IBS is less conclusive. Tricyclic agents appear modestly effective in relieving abdominal pain and diarrhea (Jackson et al., 2000), though they may also aggravate constipation (Tally, 2004). Too few placebo-controlled trials have examined the efficacy of selective serotonin reuptake inhibitors for IBS to warrant drawing conclusions regarding their efficacy (Jailwala et al., 2000; Talley, 2004). Fibromyalgia, on the other hand, appears more responsive to antidepressants than do the other functional somatic syndromes. Tricyclics appear to lessen fibromyalgia patients' pain, fatigue, and sleep difficulties (Arnold et al., 2000). Fluoxetine, a selective serotonin reuptake inhibitor, may also provide some relief from fibromyalgia symptomatology, though results from fluoxetine trials have been less consistent than those from trials with tricyclics (Arnold et al., 2000; O'Malley et al., 2000). Three recently published, large, randomized, controlled studies suggest duloxetine and milnaciprin, reuptake inhibitors of both serotonin and norepinephrine, alleviate pain and discomfort associated with fibromyalgia (Arnold et al., 2004, 2005; Gendreau et al., 2005). At present, we are aware of no evidence supporting the long-term efficacy for any of these pharmacological agents (Carette et al., 1994).

Controlled trials have not produced convincing evidence to support the use of most other pharmacological interventions for CFS or for fibromyalgia. Studies investigating the efficacy of immunotherapy, corticosteroids, and growth hormone on CFS have been unsuccessful in producing improvement (Whiting et al., 2001). Likewise, steroids, nonsteroidal anti-inflammatories, hypnotics, and muscle relaxants appear to provide little or no relief above and beyond that of a placebo to patients suffering from fibromyalgia (Clark, Tindall, & Bennett, 1985; Drewes, Andreasen, Jennum, & Nielson, 1991; Moldofsky, Lue, Mously, Roth-Schechter, & Reynolds, 1996; Quijada-Carrera et al., 1996; Tofferi, Jackson, & O'Malley, 2004; Yunus, Masi, & Aldag, 1989b). The only group of medications that has been shown to have pain-relieving effects on fibromyalgia, other than antidepressants, is the second generation of antiepileptic agents, specifically pregabalin (Crofford et al., 2005).

Research on pharmacotherapy for IBS provides some support for the use of a few agents. Smooth-muscle relaxants, bulking agents, and anticholinergic/antispasmodic agents have not consistently outperformed placebo interventions (Jailwala et al., 2000; Klein, 1988; Talley, 2003). Loperamide, an opiate without pain-relieving qualities, appears effective in reducing diarrhea, though not in reducing abdominal pain or distension (Jailwala et al., 2000). Also, two serotonergic medications, tegaserod and alosetron, have received FDA approval for the treatment of IBS, the former for the constipation-predominant type and the latter for the diarrhea-predominant type. Alosetron, however, is available only through a restricted marketing program because it has been associated with serious gastrointestinal adverse effects. Symptom relief associated with the use of either tegaserod or alosetron seems to be relatively modest (Jailwala et al., 2000; Talley, 2003).

Summary of Pharmacotherapy for Somatization Syndromes

As a whole, data from controlled clinical trials provide consistent support for a few agents: St. John's wort (for ICD-10–defined somatization), amitriptyline and duloxetine (for fibromyalgia), and tegaserod and alosetron (for IBS). Each of these treatments appears moderately effective in reducing somatization and related symptoms. Evidence for long-term efficacy is lacking.

Psychosocial Interventions

Various psychosocial interventions have been used to treat somatization syndromes. Short-term dynamic therapy, relaxation training, exercise regimens, behavior therapy, cognitive therapy, and cognitive-behavioral therapy have been tested in controlled studies with one or more of the patient groups described above. The studies are reviewed below. A more detailed examination of this literature can be found elsewhere (Allen, Escobar, Lehrer, Gara, & Woolfolk, 2002).

Short-Term Dynamic Therapy

Psychodynamic theory has proposed that unexplained physical symptoms are produced to protect the somatizer from traumatic, frightening, and/or depressing emotional experiences. If an individual fails to process a trauma adequately, it is hypothesized, the original affect later may be converted into physical symptoms (Engel, 1959). Short-term dynamically oriented treatments that explore the stress and emotional distress associated with physical symptoms have been studied systematically with patients with IBS. In one study, a short-term dynamic therapy, aimed at "modifying maladaptive behaviour and finding new solutions to problems," resulted in significantly greater improvement in IBS symptoms than did a standard medical care treatment condition (Svedlund, Sjodin, Ottosson, & Dotevall, 1983). Differences between groups were observed after treatment as well as 1 year later. Another trial examined the efficacy of a short-term dynamic therapy aimed at helping participants explore the links between IBS symptoms and emotional factors (Guthrie, Creed, Dawson, & Tomenson, 1991). The treatment was supplemented by audiotape-administered relaxation methods that participants were instructed to use at home. Immediately after the 3-month intervention phase, participants receiving psychotherapy reported significantly greater improvements in IBS symptoms than did participants receiving standard medical care. This second intervention (psychodynamic therapy plus relaxation training) was more recently compared with pharmacotherapy using paroxetine and to standard medical care for IBS. Although there were no differences among the three treatment conditions in patient-reported abdominal pain, both dynamic therapy and paroxetine were associated with greater improvement in physical functioning than was standard medical care a year after treatment. Furthermore, psychotherapy, but not paroxetine, was associated with greater reductions in healthcare costs during the year after treatment (Creed et al., 2003).

Relaxation Training

Psychophysiologists have described several mechanisms that produce somatic symptoms in the absence of organic pathology (Clauw, 1995; Gardner & Bass, 1989). These mechanisms include overactivity or dysregulation of the autonomic nervous system, smooth-muscle contractions, endocrine overactivity, and hyperventilation. Miscellaneous techniques directed at reducing physiological arousal and physical discomfort associated with unexplained physical symptoms have been studied within controlled experimental designs. Small studies have shown that relaxation techniques such as electromyogram (EMG) biofeedback and guided imagery reduce pain associated with fibromyalgia more effectively than do sham relaxation treatments (Ferraccioli et al., 1987; Fors, Sexton, & Gotestam, 2002). In another small trial, patients treated with progressive muscle relaxation reported greater relief in their irritable bowel symptoms than did patients in a control comparison treatment condition (Blanchard, Greene, Scharff, & Schwarz-McMorris, 1993).

Hypnotherapy designed to produce generalized relaxation and control of intestinal activity has been successfully applied to IBS as well as to fibromyalgia. In three different studies, hypnotherapy was associated with less abdominal pain and fewer abnormal bowel habits than was either of two comparison conditions, supportive psychotherapy combined with a placebo pill (Whorwell, Prior, & Farragher, 1984) or a symptom-monitoring condition (Galovski & Blanchard, 1998; Palsson, Turner, Johnson, Burnett, & Whitehead, 2002). The one study assessing the efficacy of hypnotherapy for fibromyalgia found it was associated with greater pain relief than was physical therapy (Haanen et al., 1991). In an attempt to examine the mechanism of improvement, Palsson and colleagues (2002) showed that improvements seen in IBS symptoms after hypnotherapy were related to improvements in somatization and in anxiety but not related to physiological measures of rectal pain threshold, rectal smooth-muscle tone, or autonomic functioning.

Exercise Treatments

Exercise interventions have been developed for somatizers in accordance with evidence suggesting that exercise improves mood, pain thresholds, and sleep (Minor, 1991; Weyerer & Kupfer, 1994). One theory explaining the benefits of exercise proposes that it produces increases in serum levels of beta-endorphin-like immunoreactivity, adrenocorticotropic hormone, prolactin, and growth hormone (Harber & Sutton, 1984). In most studies, graded exercise treatments have been associated with improvements in physical functioning, fatigue, and global well-being in patients diagnosed with CFS or fibromyalgia (Fulcher & White, 1997; Martin et al., 1996; McCain, Bell, Mai, & Halliday, 1988; Powell, Bentall, Nye, & Edwards, 2001; Richards & Scott, 2002). Some trials have even shown exercise to outperform relaxation and/or stretching comparison interventions (Fulcher & White, 1997; Martin et al., 1996; McCain et al., 1988; Richards & Scott, 2002). Although both statistically and clinically significant gains have been reported, the findings reported above probably are not generalizable to all patients with CFS or fibromyalgia. First, some investigators have not found an association between exercise treatments and symptom relief (King, Wessel, Bhambhani, Sholter, & Maksymowych, 2002; Mengshoel, Komnaes, & Forre, 1992). Second, many patients are disinclined to exercise and, thus, are unlikely to enroll in exercise studies. Finally, some studies have produced high attrition rates (Martin et al., 1996; Wearden et al., 1998), indicating that even patients who agree to undergo an exercise regimen may not adhere to it.

Behavior Therapy

Operant behavior therapy manipulates the consequences of patients' illness behavior with the aim of alleviating the associated pain and impairment (Fordyce, 1976). Recipients of operant behavior therapy are rewarded as they display "healthy behaviors" and increase activity levels. Such increases in activity are expected to result in positive interactions with the outside world, experiences of joy, and a sense of productivity. Pain behaviors, such as taking medication, wincing, complaining, and seeking treatment, are identified, labeled, and consequated. A recent study compared the efficacy of an inpatient operant behavioral treatment to that of an inpatient physical therapy for fibromyalgia (Thieme, Gromnica-Ihle, & Flor, 2003). Operant behavior therapy was conducted in groups of five to seven patients for 5 weeks. Immediately after treatment, as well as 6 and 15 months after treatment, behavior therapy was associated with substantial reductions in pain intensity, use of medication, and physician visits (Thieme et al., 2003). The only other randomized, controlled study of behavior therapy for a somatization-spectrum disorder was conducted with outpatients diagnosed with IBS. In this study, patients who received 6–15 sessions of individual behavior therapy reported no more improvement than did control participants (Corney, Stanton, Newell, Clare, & Fairclough, 1991). Discrepancies in findings from these two studies may be related to differences in patient populations (fibromyalgia vs. IBS) or interventions (inpatient, group vs. outpatient, individual). Additional research on the efficacy of behavior therapy for functional somatic syndromes is required before such interventions can be endorsed.

Cognitive Therapy

Cognitive therapy focuses on and attempts to alter faulty thinking patterns associated with functional somatic symptoms. Three trials with IBS patients have shown individual cognitive therapy to be associated with greater reductions in IBS symptoms than either a wait-list control condition or a support group (Greene & Blanchard, 1994; Payne & Blanchard, 1994; Vollmer & Blanchard, 1998). Cognitive therapy also has been shown in controlled trials to reduce the health anxiety of hypochondriacal patients (Clark et al., 1998; Visser & Bouman, 2001).

Cognitive-Behavioral Therapy

Cognitive-behavioral therapy (CBT) aims to alter dysfunctional thoughts and behaviors associated with somatization symptoms. With IBS patients, CBT usually has included a relaxation component. Controlled trials of CBT interventions for IBS have produced inconsistent results. Five trials showed CBT administered individually relieved bowel symptoms more effectively than did standard medical care (Heymann-Monnikes et al., 2000; Shaw et al., 1991), an educational attention-control condition (Drossman et al., 2003), or a wait-list (Lynch & Zamble, 1989; Neff & Blanchard, 1987). In a sixth study, CBT administered as a group treatment resulted in greater improvements in

IBS symptoms than did a wait-list control condition (Van Dulmen, Fennis, & Bleijenberg, 1996). Four other investigations found no difference between individual CBT and a control condition (Bennett & Wilkinson, 1985; Blanchard et al., 1992; Boyce, Talley, Balaam, Koloski, & Truman, 2003).

Studies of CBT for IBS have not yielded a consistent pattern of results. Discrepancies in the earlier research were, perhaps, to be expected, given its lack of methodological rigor, but the findings of two recently published and methodologically sound studies on CBT for IBS also are not congruent (Boyce et al., 2003; Drossman et al., 2003). Identifiable differences between the more recent studies' designs and outcome measures potentially provide some insight into the discrepancies in findings. Whereas Drossman and colleagues (2003) found CBT more effective than an educational intervention, Boyce and colleagues (2003) found CBT no more effective than an 8-week relaxation treatment. Because Boyce's comparison treatment condition, a relaxation intervention, has been demonstrated in past studies to reduce IBS symptoms (Blanchard et al., 1993), it was likely to have been more efficacious than was Drossman's control condition. Drossman and colleagues' primary outcome measure was a composite of the following variables: satisfaction with treatment, global well-being, abdominal pain scores from diaries, and health-related quality of life. Boyce and colleagues, on the other hand, measured outcome with the Bowel Symptom Severity Scale, a measure of frequency, disability, and distress caused by each of eight gastrointestinal symptoms. Treatment satisfaction and global well-being were not assessed in the Boyce study. The results of these two studies suggest CBT may help patients with IBS cope with their symptoms and with their lives better than do educational sessions, but may not relieve specific IBS symptoms any better than relaxation treatments.

When CBT has been administered to patients with CFS, it has not included relaxation training. Instead, encouragement to increase activities, including exercise, has been a key component of these interventions. In one study, CBT was no more effective than the control treatment (Lloyd et al., 1993), whereas in three other studies CBT reduced fatigue significantly more than did relaxation (Deale, Chalder, Marks, & Wessely, 1997), support groups (Prins et al., 2001), or standard medical care (Sharpe et al., 1996). One study found the superiority of CBT over relaxation to be maintained 5 years after treatment (Deale, Kaneez, Chalder, & Wessely, 2001). The trials that found CBT to be efficacious employed more intensive treatments than did the one unsuccessful trial. The clinical impact achieved in the successful trials, coupled with the methodological quality of the trials, lends further support to the use of CBT with patients with CFS.

For fibromyalgia, the efficacy of group CBT, but not of individually administered CBT, has been studied in controlled trials with fibromyalgia patients. Patients treated with a six-session group CBT reported significantly greater improvement in physical functioning, but not in pain, 12 months after baseline when compared with patients who had received standard medical care (Williams et al., 2002). Another trial, comparing the efficacy of a group CBT to that of group relaxation training (autogenic training), showed no differences between the conditions at posttreatment, but 4 months later, CBT participants reported a greater reduction in pain intensity than did the autogenic training participants (Keel, Bodoky, Gerhard, & Muller, 1998). Two trials comparing a CBT/education group with a discussion/education group found no difference in pain complaints or functioning between the two treatment conditions (Nicassio et al., 1997; Vlaeyen et al., 1996). The findings of a less than powerful impact of CBT on fibromyalgia may reflect the ineffectiveness of group-administered treatment for this population. The benefits of individual CBT have yet to be explored with patients with fibromyalgia.

Investigators have conducted controlled treatment trials assessing the efficacy of CBT with patients complaining of at least one unexplained medical symptom. In one study, patients treated with individual CBT showed greater improvement in their psychosomatic complaints than did patients treated with standard medical care (Speckens et al., 1995). Another study found group CBT superior to a wait-list control condition in reducing physical symptoms and hypochondriacal beliefs (Lidbeck, 1997). In both studies, improvements were observed after treatment as well as 6 months later (Lidbeck, 1997; Speckens et al., 1995). Lidbeck's CBT participants seemed to maintain reductions in somatization and hypochondriacal beliefs 18 months after treatment (Lidbeck, 2003). Two other studies demonstrated reductions in the health anxiety of pure-hypochondriasis patients treated with CBT (Barsky & Ahern, 2004; Warwick, Clark, Cobb, & Salkovskis, 1996).

Three studies have examined the efficacy of individually administered CBT with patients manifesting a diverse set of unexplained physical symptoms. Two studies were conducted in primary care settings with patients who were diagnosed with subthreshold somatization, defined as abridged somatization in one study (Escobar et al., 2006) and defined as five or more unexplained physical symptoms in the other (Sumathipala, Hewege, Hanwella, & Mann, 2000). The third study included only patients meeting DSM-IV criteria for full somatization disorder (Allen et al., 2006). Both the Allen and colleagues (2006) and the Escobar and colleagues (2006) studies followed the treatment manual outlined in Appendix A of this book and compared standard medical care augmented by a psychiatric consultation with CBT administered in conjuction with augmented standard medical care. All three studies showed individual CBT to be associated with greater reductions in somatic complaints than were comparison conditions (Allen et al., 2006; Escobar et al., 2006; Sumathipala et al., 2000). The study examining the efficacy of CBT for full somatization disorder is described in detail in Appendix B.

Other Treatments

Two other psychosocial interventions for full somatization disorder have been subjected to empirical investigation. Smith, Monson, and Ray (1986b) sent a psychiatric consultation letter to the patients' physicians, describing somatization disorder and providing recommendations to guide primary care. The recommendations to physicians were straightforward: (1) to schedule somatizers' appointments every 4–6 weeks instead of "as needed," (2) to conduct a physical examination in the organ system or body part relevant to the presenting complaint, (3) to avoid diagnostic procedures and surgeries unless clearly indicated by underlying somatic pathology, and (4) to avoid making disparaging statements, such as "Your symptoms are all in your head." Patients whose primary physicians had received the consultation letter experienced better health outcomes (physical functioning and cost of medical care) than those whose physicians had not received the letter. The results have been replicated in two different samples of patients (Rost, Kashner, & Smith, 1994; Smith et al., 1986b; Smith, Rost, & Kashner, 1995). The second intervention included group psychotherapy encouraging emotional expression and providing peer support, coping skills, and psychoeducation. This group intervention, in combination with the above-mentioned psychiatric consultation letter, was associated with significantly greater improvements in physical functioning and mental health than occurred in the control group that received standard medical treatment augmented by the psychiatric consultation letter (Kashner, Rost, Cohen, Anderson, & Smith, 1995). The efficacy of the group therapy component of the intervention, however, is rendered uncertain due to poor attendance at treatment sessions.

Summary of Psychosocial Interventions for Somatization Syndromes

In general, psychosocial interventions have been moderately effective in reducing the physical symptoms associated with somatization-spectrum disorders. Investigators who reported long-term outcome data suggest that benefits persist as much as a year after treatment. Although detailed descriptions of most interventions are not provided in research articles, close scrutiny of the studies' methods sections suggests a great deal of overlap among the interventions. For example, one of the dynamically oriented therapies included a relaxation component. The other dynamic treatment involved directive, prescriptive interventions: encouraging patients to change maladaptive behavior and to engage in problem-solving exercises. CBT often incorporated relaxation training or homework assignments directing patients to engage in physical exercise. With so much overlap among treatments, perhaps it is not surprising that none of the interventions appears to be discernibly more potent than any of the others.

Psychosocial versus Pharmacological Treatments

A few studies have compared the efficacy of a psychosocial intervention with that of a pharmacological treatment for somatization syndromes. Patients with CFS who participated in an exercise treatment reported greater improvements in fatigue and functional capacity than did patients with CFS treated with fluoxetine (Wearden et al., 1998). Guided imagery produced results in fibromyalgia pain superior to amitriptyline (Fors et al., 2002). For IBS, both paroxetine and psychodynamic therapy were more effective in enhancing physical functioning than was standard medical care, though only psychotherapy was associated with reductions in healthcare costs (Creed et al., 2003). In an older study on IBS, Svedlund and colleagues' (1983) psychodynamic treatment outperformed the control treatment, which included physician-prescribed bulking agents, anticholingergic drugs, antacids, and minor tranquilizers. These last three studies suggest a psychosocial intervention might be more effective than the medications most frequently prescribed for fibromyalgia and IBS. Nevertheless, too few studies have included the kinds of comparisons that would justify this conclusion. Additional research is needed to examine the relative and combined efficacies of pharmacological and behavioral interventions with somatization syndromes.

It is important to note that the majority of studies reported here were conducted in controlled tertiary care settings with patients who may not be representative of the total population of individuals with somatization syndromes. All patients described in the above studies chose to participate in a research study employing a randomized, control-group design. Thus, the generalizability of findings is limited.

Whether these treatments could be exported to the arena of primary care with the same efficacy is a question for future research.

SOMATIZATION IN CHILDREN AND ADOLESCENTS

The symptom most commonly reported in pediatric primary care clinics is recurrent abdominal pain (RAP) (Fritz, Fritsch, & Hagino, 1997). Apley and Naish (1958) first used the term RAP to label three or more episodes of abdominal pain that are severe enough to interfere with activities and occur over a period of at least 3 months. RAP has been associated with significant disruptions in daily functioning, including school absenteeism (Liebman, 1978), and with anxious and depressed moods (Garber, Zeman, & Walker, 1990). Although not specified as such in the criteria for RAP, many researchers have conceptualized RAP as a functional syndrome.

Other somatization syndromes also are prevalent in children and adolescents (Campo & Fritsch, 1994; Fritz et al., 1997; Lieb et al., 2002). Approximately 10–30% of school-age children report recurrent somatic symptoms (Garber, Walker, & Zeman, 1991; Offord et al., 1987; Perquin et al., 2000). Somatization disorder, subthreshold somatization, fibromyalgia, CFS, and IBS have been reported in this age group. Because the diagnostic criteria for each of these disorders were established for adults, the use of less stringent and more developmentally appropriate criteria for juvenile subtypes has been suggested (Campo, Jansen-McWilliams, Comer, & Kelleher, 1999; Siegel, Janeway, & Baum, 1998; Walker et al., 2004).

Children and adolescents presenting with somatization syndromes share many of the characteristics of adult somatizers. Often juvenile somatizers function poorly (especially in school), overuse medical services, and report high rates of emotional distress (Campo et al., 1999). Also, their parents report high rates of somatization symptoms, as well as depression and anxiety (Garber et al., 1990; Walker, Garber, & Greene, 1991). Although a sex difference has not been observed in the occurrence of somatization syndromes in young children, adolescent girls are more likely to report somatization symptoms than are adolescent boys (Campo et al., 1999; Garber et al., 1991).

Treatment for juvenile somatization has been examined in very few controlled studies. Pediatricians have been encouraged to follow similar guidelines as those recommended for primary care physicians treating adult somatizers (e.g., Smith et al., 1986b). Specifically, they are advised to maintain a regimen of regularly scheduled check-ups, conduct physical examinations at check-ups, avoid unnecessary diagnostic or invasive treatment procedures, and focus on reducing dysfunction rather than making an overall diagnosis (Fritz et al., 1997). The efficacies of these recommendations, however, have not been studied systematically.

Controlled studies have been conducted on the efficacy of family cognitive-behavioral therapy for both RAP and CFS. These treatments have two targets: to train children and/or adolescents to use stress management techniques for their symptoms and to train their parents not to reinforce illness behavior (Robins, Smith, Glutting, & Bishop, 2005; Sanders et al., 1989; Sanders, Shepherd, Cleghorn, & Woolford, 1994; Stulemeijer, de Jong, Fiselier, Hoogveld, & Bleijenberg, 2005). These four studies suggest such interventions are moderately effective in reducing symptomatology and dysfunction.

CHAPTER 3

Affective Cognitive-Behavioral Therapy for Somatization

Rationale and Overview

Rahim was a computer programmer who had been very successful as a consultant in New York City during the 1990s. He had worked for major financial institutions and earned several hundred thousand dollars per year. The work was not always that difficult given Rahim's very high aptitude, but it entailed long hours and many deadlines. Many of his coworkers complained of stress, and a few even suggested that the pressure the work entailed was unhealthy. Rahim did not believe it. He was proud of his achievements and was regarded as something of a celebrity in his hometown in India, an example of a local boy who had made good in America. The small portion of his income that he sent home each month was a huge sum to his family in India.

Rahim started having headaches in 2000, beginning when the stock market began to fluctuate and then to go down. Rumors of a contraction in the job market provoked no feelings of fear in him, but when he found himself getting fewer calls from headhunters, he also began to experience additional symptoms that baffled his primary care physician. Rahim began to feel a burning sensation in his hands and feet. Sometimes he felt sharp pains in his joints. When his wife suggested that it must be the stress of the tech bubble bursting, Rahim really didn't know what to say. He was not an emotional person, and he was not aware of being distressed about his work or his finances.

In this chapter we describe the rationales for our treatment for somatization. We describe our therapeutic conceptualization and the premises that underlie it. We also provide a description of our overall

46

approach and discuss how it compares to and contrasts with other forms of therapy. We address, as well, the special issues raised by working with patients with somatization like Rahim and the therapeutic postures and methods that seem most appropriate and helpful.

THE MANY FACETS OF SOMATIZATION

Somatization can be viewed from a variety of perspectives. There is no unified and comprehensive scientific theory of somatization that has been verified by empirical research. Notwithstanding, we do subscribe, tentatively, to a multifaceted model of the disorder, each component of which has received support in the empirical literature. This model informs and guides our therapeutic efforts to ameliorate the discomfort and disability of individuals with unexplained medical symptoms. An underlying tenet of the model is perhaps an axiom of the biopsychosocial view of medical phenomena. The problems that people bring to healers can be understood at many levels: biochemical, physiological, psychological, cultural, and societal. Somatization, being a particularly perplexing mind–brain–body kind of problem, is especially resistant to unitary explanations. Our model of somatization has four foci, four categories of explanation that involve somewhat different levels of analysis and that address most aspects of the biopsychosocial framework: the biological, psychological, behavioral, and sociocultural. The categories we employ are not theoretically distinct. In fact, they clearly overlap somewhat and are in some instances complementary. What follows is an attempt to articulate the essentials of each.

Stress

There are many standard accounts of how psychosocial stress can act as a contributing factor in a variety of somatic and mental disorders. With respect to somatization, stress typically has been regarded as a pivotal, if not a primary, etiological factor. There is a research literature supporting this view and also a medical habit of mind and locution that automatically implicates stress when disease processes are not well understood and have not been specified. In this latter circumstance, the term "stress" can serve as a proxy for all kinds of environmental influences and psychological reactions. Often, stress and emotional factors are implicated in concert. Some writers, indeed, define stress as the organism's psychophysiological response to threatening or perturbing circumstances, blurring the boundary between stress and emotion. Although our own inclination is to refer to stress as a stimulus rather than a response, emotion and the organismic response to stressors overlap extensively in our account. Given that the discourses on stress and emotion come from different traditions, emphasize different features, and use somewhat different terminology, it is rhetorically useful to separate them in our discussion.

The immediate somatic changes that occur in response to psychosocial stress are well known. The hypothalamus directly enervates fibers of the sympathetic nervous system, causing the adrenal medulla to secrete epinephrine and norepinephrine into the bloodstream, producing elevations in breathing rate, heart rate, blood pressure, and blood glucose, as well as "deactivating" the digestive system. This coordinated set of responses is the immediate disruption of homeostasis that makes the body more effective in coping with various environmental events; it is sometimes referred to as the adrenomedullary response. A second, longer-term response associated with the hypothalamic–pituitary–adrenal (HPA) axis results when the hypothalamus secretes corticotropin-releasing hormone (CRH) into the hypothalamic–pituitary circulatory system, triggering release of adrenocorticotropic hormone (ACTH) by the anterior pituitary. ACTH travels through the bloodstream to the adrenal glands, where it stimulates the production and release of glucocorticoids (e.g., cortisol) and mineralocorticoids (e.g., aldosterone) by the adrenal cortex. Glucocorticoids have widespread and complex effects, as all cells in the body have glucocorticoid receptors. In most cases, glucocorticoids remain elevated during chronic stress and have been implicated as proximate causes for a number of potentially pathogenic processes, such as the attenuation of inflammation and suppression of specific immunity.

The effect of stress on bodily organs involves many complicated feedback systems that only now are beginning to be understood. As an example, the body possesses complex machinery for cortisol secretion and regulation of cortisol levels circulating in the blood. Once cortisol rises to threshold levels after a stressful event, mechanisms of negative feedback inhibition begin to down-regulate the pituitary's production of ACTH, ultimately reducing plasma cortisol levels. This feedback loop has been implicated in various confusing and contradictory findings regarding cortisol in populations that have been subjected to severe stress. Patients with posttraumatic stress disorder (PTSD) appear to have subnormal blood levels of cortisol, although one might predict cortisol to be elevated in this population (Yehuda, 1997). Recent research has suggested that this finding is the result of a recalibration of the HPA axis such that the mechanism of ACTH secretion is so sensitized to the presence of cortisol that the cortisol-producing mechanism quickly overloads and shuts itself off (Yehuda, Golier, Halligan, Meaney, & Bierer, 2004). Bidirectional feedback loops also exist between the gut and the brain along what is sometimes referred to as the brain–gut axis, the direct and indirect mechanisms of information exchange between the gastrointestinal system and the central nervous system. The vagus nerve not only transmits signals from the brain to initiate such processes as peristalsis (mediated via parasympathetic enervation), but also sends information from the gut to the brain. Through direct neural linkages that bypass the cortex, information processing within the emotion centers of the brain may have direct impact on sensations in the gastrointestinal system, and sensations in the gut may also feed back into the brain, affecting its emotional processing centers. Unpleasant sensations from the gut may cause distress and discomfort not only via the standard mechanisms involved in the conscious perception of discomfort but also through vagally mediated subcortical processes. Pleasant sensations, such as satiety, also may have direct effects on the brain through mechanisms that bypass awareness. Functional gastrointestinal disorders may result from stress but also can function themselves as stressors.

There is increasing evidence of abnormalities in the stress systems of patients with somatization, specifically in sensory processing and HPA axis functioning. Investigators have found a hyperreactivity to high-intensity stimuli. For example, excessive augmentation of sensory evoked potentials has been reported in patients diagnosed with somatization disorder, psychogenic pain, chronic pain, or hysterical anesthesia as compared with control research participants (James, Gordon, Kraiuhin, Howson, & Meares, 1990; Moldofsky & England, 1975; Mushin & Levy, 1974; von Knorring, Almay, Johansson, & Terenius, 1979). Consistent with these results, Bushbaum (1975) demonstrated that individuals with high pain tolerances have reduced evoked potentials. Other studies have found patients with fibromyalgia to be no more accurate in detecting electrical pressure or thermal stimulation, but rather to consider such stimuli as painful or unpleasant at lower levels than do control participants (Arroyo & Cohen, 1993; Lautenbacher, Rollman, & McCain, 1994). Also, Rief, Shaw, and Fichter (1998) found that patients presenting with somatization have higher levels of physiological arousal and are less likely to habituate to a stressful task than control subjects. HPA axis dysfunction, as evidenced by reduced levels of circulating cortisol, has been observed in patients diagnosed with chronic fatigue syndrome (CFS) (Cleare et al., 1999; Demitrack et al., 1991), idiopathic pain (Alfven, de la Torre, & Uvnas-Moberg, 1994; Johansson, 1982; Valdes, Garcia, Treserra, de Pablo, & de

Flores, 1989; Von Knorring & Almay, 1989), and chronic headache (Elwan, Abdella, el Bayad, & Hamdy, 1991).

The response to stress is complex, involving many mechanisms that are not fully understood, and there are intergender and inter-individual variations (Taylor et al., 2000). Despite our inability to delineate many features of the causal process, we know that protracted activation of the stress response is, for the most part, pathogenic. This wear and tear on the body produced by chronic stress is termed "allostatic load" (McEwen, 2005). Various subtle, widespread, and complex disruptions of somatic systems result from prolonged stress. Specific immunity and inflammation operate less effectively, the cardiovascular system is taxed, the gastrointestinal system is perturbed, and muscular tension is increased. Stress can produce or exacerbate many prototypical somatization symptoms, among them headaches (Ehde & Holm, 1992), noncardiac chest pain (Anderson, Dalton, Bradley, & Richter, 1989), and gastrointestinal (GI) symptoms (Locke, Weaver, Melton, & Talley, 2004; Whitehead, Crowell, Robinson, Heller, & Schuster, 1992). In addition, recent research in animals has demonstrated a stress-induced hyperalgesia in rats (King, Devine, Vierck, Rodgers, & Yezierski, 2003), a finding consistent with anecdotal reports that stress increases clinical pain in humans.

Within the research literature, stress has been defined and operationalized in many ways. Among these are exposure to combat, experience of a natural disaster, disruptive life change, difficult workplace environment, physical abuse, daily "hassles," and many others. The established relationship between such stressful circumstances and physical symptoms has been reported on occasions far too numerous to review in a book that is focused on therapeutic intervention rather than experimental psychopathology. Despite some methodological shortcomings and ambiguities in results, it is safe to conclude that stress contributes to the occurrence of medically unexplained physical symptoms. An association between stress and physical symptoms has been shown for natural disasters (Lindeman, Saari, Verkasalo, & Prytz, 1996), warfare (Neria & Koenen, 2003; Soetekouw et al., 2000), vocational demands (Frese, 1999), daily "hassles" (DeLongis, Folkman, & Lazarus, 1988), and academic pressures (Takata, 2001).

Although theory and research on psychosocial stress and somatization must be considered preliminary, much data and current psychophysiological theory implicate stress as a contributory factor in somatization. In addition, treatment methods effective in reducing the impact of stress also appear to have therapeutic impact on some cases of somatization (see Chapter 2). Techniques of stress management, therefore, are central features of our treatment program.

Emotion

Had this book been written a quarter of a century ago, quite possibly very little mention of emotion might have been made. At the height of the cognitive revolution, emotions were widely regarded as feeling states that derived exclusively from cognitive appraisals. Zajonc's (1980) seminal paper challenged cognitivist views of emotion and demonstrated that emotional responses are, at least partially, independent of cognition and may occur unconsciously. Emotion theorist Paul Ekman (1992) has argued for an "automatic appraisal mechanism" that is faster than cognition and provides a rapid evaluative response to the environment. More recent research (LeDoux, 1996) has shown not only that some emotional reactions (e.g., fear) can be elicited independent of conscious thought processes, but also that there are neural pathways that channel information directly into the amygdala without its first passing through the neocortex, where processing must occur for the affect to attain consciousness. Two studies (Whalen et al., 1998, 2004) found that brief, backward masked presentations of pictures of fearful, as compared with happy, faces activated the amygdala even though participants were unaware that either type of face had been presented. A similar study found that behaviorally relevant features in the visual environment can be detected and processed without conscious awareness, via a colliculo–pulvinar–amygdalar pathway of activation that controls reflexive and autonomic responses and bypasses the cortex (Morris, Ohman, & Dolan, 1999).

Our brains process sensory input at a variety of levels. One of these levels involves the everyday, common-sense picture of information processing wherein a stimulus occurs and we consciously perceive it, cognitively interpret it, and are aware of a mood state associated with it. Recent research, however, suggests that sometimes stimuli are perceived without awareness, resulting in an unconscious "emotional" response, one that may affect the body in the same way as a conscious feeling state. Much contemporary research in social psychology has shown that attitudes, prejudices, and stereotypes can be evoked and can influence behavior without the associated processes ever entering awareness (Bargh & Chartrand, 1999). In a similar fashion, human beings can have emotional reactions that affect their bodies, but that occur outside of awareness, in what amounts to subsymbolic information processing or, as some would put it, implicit or unconscious affect (Winkielman & Berridge, 2004). Current theory suggests that humans become conscious of an emotional response to a stimulus only if that response receives interpretation in the cortex. Thus, contemporary views of emotion incorporate a kind of unconscious emotional processing analogous to that posited by psychoanalysis and various forms of psychodynamic psychotherapy, but that is not emphasized by cognitive-behavioral therapists. From the pop psychology of emotional intelligence to the neuroscience of appetitive and defensive reactions, the existence and significance of unconscious emotional reactions to the environment are very much at the center of contemporary science.

Emotions are properly conceived as brain processes, some conscious and some unconscious, at times affecting the body just as stress does. Emotional processing can and does occur without awareness. In the case of certain defensive reactions (e.g., fear) the accounts are straightforward and helpfully informed by animal models. Human beings who are frightened in everyday life have a great deal in common physiologically with infrahumans who are threatened with harmful stimuli in the laboratory. The full spectrum of human emotions, however, is manifold and complex, and we are very far from fully understanding all the various ways emotions interact with somatic systems. Early research results suggest that emotions are palpable and significant influences on health. Negative emotions and moods have been linked to various forms of disease and discomfort (Greenwood, Thurston, Rumble, Waters, & Keefe, 2003; Linton, 2000; O'Leary, 1990; Todaro et al., 2003). Positive emotions, on the other hand, are associated with longevity and favorable health outcomes (Danner, Snowdon, & Friesen, 2001; Fredrickson & Levenson, 1998).

Although the mediators of the effects of the emotions on health and health on the emotions are only dimly understood, much has been learned in recent years. Again the gastrointestinal system provides a useful illustration. The influence of the emotions upon GI function has been assumed for centuries, but only recently has empirical research begun to describe its specific contours. In the case of functional GI disorders the emotions appear to be involved in a cause–effect loop that is illustrated by the reciprocal interaction between bodily systems and emotion centers in the brain. The emotional expressions of fear (Welgan, Meshkinpour, & Hoehler, 1985) and anger (Welgan, Meshkinpour, & Beeler, 1988) as well as the tendency to suppress anger (Evans, Bennett, Bak, Tennent, & Kellow, 1996) are associated with elevated gastric motility. Mayer, Naliboff, and Chang (2001) suggest that the response of the GI system to the emotions may exhibit a degree of specificity. These authors report that fear is associated with inhibition of upper GI (stomach and duodenum) contractions and secretions and with stimulation of lower GI (sigmoid colon and rectum) motility and secretions. The first may produce the feeling of fullness and the absence of appetite, while the second may lead to lower bowel pain and to diarrhea. It may be that this response pattern of the digestive tract evolved in order to minimize the exposure of the intestines to ingested food and waste material during a time when bodily resources need to be directed toward the skeletomotor system to enhance coping with threatening physical events. With the emotion of anger, the pattern of upper GI activity is transposed, with the production of acid secretion and gastric contractions. Thus, depending on the specific emotional context (fear vs. anger), the upper GI tract will be either inhibited (fear) or stimulated (anger). Mayer, Naliboff, and Munakata (2000) also present evidence that responses of the viscera produce autonomic output that is fed back to the brain, affecting conscious and unconscious emotional processes. Recent studies using brain imaging methodology have demonstrated activation of the brain's emotion-processing centers following artificial stimulation of the gut, even when that stimulation is subliminal (Hamaguchi et al., 2004; Kern & Shaker, 2002).

The implications of contemporary emotion theory and the findings presented above resonate with the older clinical literature, some of it dating back to the Renaissance, suggesting that somatization results from suppressed, blocked, partially expressed, or unexperienced emotion. In a sense the "idioms of distress" literature, inspired by cross-cultural research, has a very similar model of somatization (i.e., implicit emotion being expressed through physical distress and suffering). The empirical research that has addressed the relationship between emotion and somatization contains various methodological weaknesses. Although that literature does not paint a simple picture of the relationship between emotion and somatization, it does suggest that the two are related in important and complex ways. One set of findings suggests that individuals who do not readily experience the full range of affects are susceptible to experience medically unexplained symptoms.

"Alexithymia," a term coined by psychoanalyst Peter E. Sifneos (1973), literally means having no words for emotions or feelings. Nemiah, Freyberger, and Sifneos (1976) posited alexithymia to involve several features: difficulty in identifying subjective feelings, difficulty in describing feelings to others, and an externally oriented cognitive style that directs focus away from one's inner experience. According to the theory, patients with alexithymia may label themselves as depressed or anxious, but their access to and reporting of specific affects will be minimal or impoverished; they will describe their experience in nebulous language, reporting such inner states as boredom, agitation, restlessness, and tension (Taylor, Bagby, & Parker, 1997). Alexithymia has been implicated in somatization by various theorists.

Their claims can be reduced essentially to the presumed somatization/ psychologization contrast and incompatibility of the two processes. If somatization is the antithesis of psychologization, as the argument goes, somatizers should score high on measures that assess how "out of touch" they are with their emotions.

The most widely studied measure of alexithymia is the Toronto Alexithymia Scale (the TAS and its newer version, the TAS-20; Bagby, Parker, & Taylor, 1994; Bagby, Taylor, & Parker, 1994; Taylor, Bagby, Ryan, & Parker, 1990). The TAS-20 is a 20-item self-report scale that has been found to be multidimensional in factor-analytic studies. The subscales of the TAS-20 correspond to three aspects of the alexithymia construct: TAS-DIF, difficulty in identifying feelings and in distinguishing between emotions and bodily sensations; TAS-DDF, difficulty describing feelings to others; and TAS-EOT, externally oriented thinking.

Despite some inconsistencies in results and some questions about the validity of the TAS as a measure of the construct of alexithymia, the TAS does show moderate levels of positive correlation with somatization. Although Lundh and Simonsson-Sarnecki (2001) found the relationship between alexithymia and somatization to be weak and accounted for by the association between alexithymia and neuroticism, two methodologically sophisticated studies (Deary, Scott, & Wilson, 1997; Waller & Scheidt, 2006) found that alexithymia accounted for unique variance in medically unexplained symptoms even when the effects of neuroticism were removed statistically. Two recent reviews have cast further doubt upon the psychometrics of the TAS but have upheld the conclusion that alexithymia is likely a contributory factor in somatization (De Gucht & Heiser, 2003; Sayar & Ak, 2001). De Gucht and Heiser's (2003) review concluded that the TAS-DIF subscale is moderately positively correlated with the number of physical symptoms endorsed on a symptom questionnaire, the TAS-DDF has a small positive correlation with symptom reporting, and the TAS-EOT is unrelated to symptom reporting. Although studies that examine the association between somatization and the construct of alexithymia as assessed by the self-report TAS need to be supplemented by studies of somatization and the construct of alexithymia measured by other means of assessment, such as a structured interview, there is considerable evidence from both clinical impressions and empirical research that many somatizers have poor ability to experience and articulate their affect.

Another body of research has studied "repressive coping," a construct that has been compared to alexithymia, given that, in both, attenuated reports of experienced affect are observed (Lane, Sechrest, Reidel, Shapiro, & Kaszniak, 2000). Repressive coping is assessed via a measure originally designed to assess the construct of social desirability, a tendency to respond in accord with social norms on self-report inventories, the Marlowe–Crowne scale (MC; Crowne & Marlowe, 1960). Individuals who score high on the MC and also score low on measures of negative affect, especially measures of anxiety, are then defined as high on repressive coping. Repressive coping is conceptualized as resulting from some as yet unspecified process of psychological defense, evoking resonances with original psychodynamic formulations of repressed emotions. Although it is not clear what mechanism underlies repressive coping, recent research suggests that repressive copers are self-deceivers rather than individuals who are aware of their affect and simply fail to report it (Derakshan & Eysenck, 1999). The overall body of evidence, though not completely coherent and homogeneous, suggests that individuals who are not aware of and do not express affect may actually experience heightened physiological responses to stress and concomitant subsymbolic emotional processing of experience. In experiments in which participants were subjected to psychological stress (giving a speech), repressive copers showed high physiological reactivity and elevated behavioral signs of anxiety, even though they reported low levels of anxious affect (Newton & Contrada, 1992). Research demonstrates that repressive coping is associated with compromised immune system function (Jamner, Schwartz, & Leigh, 1988), stress-related increases in blood pressure (King, Taylor, Albright, & Haskell, 1990), pain severity among chronic pain patients (Deshields, Tait, Gfeller, & Chibnall, 1995), and irritable bowel symptoms (Toner, Koyama, Garfinkel, & Jeejeebhoy, 1992).

If there is one clinical stereotype of the somatizer, that of the stoic, tight-lipped, defensive, overcontrolled, uncommunicative individual obsessed with her body, there also is another: that of the neurotic, hypersensitive, histrionic person, with comorbid anxiety and depression, who dramatically verbalizes one complaint after another, in both the psychological and somatic domains. The empirical literature, although presenting a nebulous and sometimes inconsistent picture, also supports this latter picture of the patient with somatization, a picture that is ostensibly inconsistent with the alexithymic, defensive image. The research literature shows high comorbidity of somatization on the one hand and the affective and anxiety disorders on the other (Tomasson, Kent, & Coryell, 1991). As a group, somatizers also score very high on measures of neuroticism, indicating that they experience much negative affect (Deary et al., 1997; Russo, Katon, Sullivan, Clark, & Buchwald, 1994).

What are we to make of this somewhat contradictory set of findings, some of which suggest that somatizers need to get in touch with their feelings and others that suggest that they have a surfeit of negative affect that needs to be attenuated, controlled, and made less toxic? We find in our clinical work that both views are true, that both stereotypes correspond to real patients we encounter. Moreover, sometimes both defensive and histrionic tendencies can exist within the same person at different times and places and in relation to different psychological issues. Our own view of somatizers is that they have various difficulties in emotional processing, difficulties that can exist side by side, each of which can generate physical symptoms. In the terms of a recently proposed theory, one might say that among somatizers we observe various forms of emotional dysregulation involving emotional valence, emotional intensity/regulation, and emotional disconnection (Berenbaum, Raghavan, Le, Vernon, & Gomez, 2003). We often find that the affect reported or displayed by somatizers seems incongruent with eliciting circumstances, being either disproportionately minimal on the one hand or negative and exaggerated on the other.

Our early work with somatizers using a standard cognitive-behavioral therapy (CBT) approach, identifying and challenging cognitions associated with physical and affective experiences, proved to have some limitations. Somatizers are simply too out of touch too much of the time with experience that must be accessed as a prerequisite for identifying dysfunctional cognitions. Thus, we have aimed to design a treatment that helps patients access and process their implicit cognitive and emotional responses. The approach involves a constant tacking between emotions and cognitions. We seek not only, in the vein of CBT, to identify and alter dysfunctional cognition so as to attenuate excessive negative affect, but also to employ a thorough cultivation and exploration of affect as a means of helping patients better understand their cognitions and their behavior. Our explorations of patients' thoughts and feelings that are related to their physical symptoms are designed, in part, to teach and encourage patients to express themselves emotionally and to reduce defensiveness. We also train our patients to develop more sensitive powers of proprioception. Helping patients tune into their internal sensations and interpret those sensations accurately is a goal of our treatment. We hypothesize that incomplete or distorted emotional processing in a sense deprives individuals of data that is important for effective problem solving and decision making. Poor understanding of the emotional domain also may result in unresolved negative affective states and in a prolongation of the physiological arousal that accompanies negative affect.

Fortunately, there is a wealth of therapeutic technique to draw upon in this area. Traditionally, psychotherapy has been, in some sense, a vehicle for people to gain access to their emotions and to become somewhat accepting of their affective responses to the world. In our work with emotion, we draw heavily upon humanistic psychotherapy, especially the practices of person-centered therapy (Rogers, 1961) and Gestalt therapy (Perls, 1973). Most therapists these days do a bit of "active listening" with their clients and attempt to foster some features of the kind of empathic, supportive, genuine interpersonal relationship that Rogers advocated. But with the proliferation of active, directive, brief modes of treatment, thorough exploration and careful listening to patients has come to be less emphasized than in days gone by, when listening perhaps was considered to be the core competency of the psychotherapist (Reik, 1948). The techniques of Gestalt therapy are unsurpassed as devices for accessing affect. They have been experiencing a bit of a revival in the very creative work of Leslie Greenberg and his colleagues on emotion-focused therapy (Greenberg, 2002; Greenberg & Watson, 2005), work that has influenced aspects of our approach to patients.

Cognition, Behavior, and Social Learning Theory

A cognitive-behavioral conceptualization emphasizes the role that patterns of cognition and behavior and contingencies of reinforcement play in the etiology and maintenance of somatic symptoms. The cognitive-behavioral approach has various historical antecedents. Operant and classical conditioning theory and research have provided models of the acquisition and retention of behavioral patterns that were adopted by the behavior therapy movement and applied to psychiatric patients. The confluence of behavior therapy and those cognitive approaches to psychotherapy espoused by Aaron Beck (1976) and Albert Ellis (1962) yielded what we recognize as our contemporary cognitive-behavioral therapy. CBT is the most extensively researched form of psychotherapy, the one that has achieved the strongest empirical support, and the approach most commonly regarding as exemplifying the ideals of evidence-based medicine.

From cognitive psychology came the view that cognitive appraisals are central to both psychological stress and human emotion. As we have seen, however, the degree to which the organism's response to environmental vicissitudes is mediated by the associative cortex (versus via less evolutionarily advanced mechanisms that operate subsymbolically) has been a matter of controversy and has been subject to some revision since the high-water mark of cognitive influence on the psychology of emotion. Cognitive-behavioral models of such disorders as depression, panic disorder, phobia, and obsessive–compulsive disorder have been extraordinarily influential and have been associated with significant psychotherapeutic advances. Some of these models have been applied and adapted for the explanation of somatization.

Many somatizers have distorted, illogical, or false beliefs. Some believe that they are physically quite fragile, even that they are mortally ill, despite evidence to the contrary (Rief, Hiller, & Margraf, 1998). Many possess the kinds of primary appraisals that have been found to be associated with and to generate negative affectivity. In addition, patients with somatization form negative cognitive appraisals of their benign physical sensations (Rief, Hiller, & Margraf, 1998). Many believe that pain, fatigue, or discomfort of any kind is a sign of disease. In addition to misinterpreting somatic sensations, some patients with somatization think catastrophically to the extent that they may consider persistent physical sensations as evidence that they suffer from a potentially fatal disease, such as cancer or AIDS (Hiller, Rief, & Fichter, 2002).

Barsky, Wyshak, and Klerman (1990) described a cognitive style of somatosensory amplification as the core aspect of a cognitive-behavioral model for hypochondriasis and demonstrated significant differences between hypochondriacal and control participants on the somatosensory amplification scale. Barsky, Coeytaux, Sarnie, and Cleary (1993) demonstrated that hypochondriacal patients believed good health to be a relatively symptom-free state and considered symptoms to be equivalent to sickness. This kind of inaccurate, irrational concept of health could contribute to a perceptual and cognitive style of somatosensory amplification wherein minor deviations from optimal functioning or comfort are interpreted as signs of disease (Salkovskis & Warwick, 2001). Recently Rief, Hiller, and Margraf (1998) presented data indicating that some cognitive patterns previously observed in patients with hypochondriasis also occur in patients with unexplained medical symptoms. In this study, patients with multiple somatization symptoms exhibited tendencies toward catastrophic interpretation of minor somatic complaints. These patients also saw themselves as lacking in robustness and believed themselves to be unable to tolerate stress.

Behavior, cognition, and emotion can interact in complex patterns, sometimes forming vicious, pathogenic circles. Dysfunctional cognitions elicit negative emotions and foster maladaptive behaviors. Thoughts of possible illness give rise to feelings of anxiety, dysphoria, and frustration, which are likely to generate and maintain physiological arousal and physical symptomatology and, hence, be interpreted as further evidence of serious illness or fragility. This physiological arousal is compounded by a tendency to amplify somatosensory information, to form negative cognitive appraisals of physical sensations, and to think catastrophically, in that persistent physical sensations are misinterpreted as signs of a potentially fatal disease. Techniques of CBT have focused for the most part either on manipulation of contingencies of reinforcement or on restructuring cognitions so as to eliminate or attenuate negative affect. Such techniques would likely be efficacious in the treatment of disorders that are characterized by negative affect and pathogenic contingencies of reinforcement. As seen in Chapter 2, the literature has supported the use of CBT with functional somatic syndromes.

From an operant conditioning perspective there are various potential "payoffs" associated with somatization. Somatizers seek comfort from those around them. Complaints and expressions of distress can be conceptualized as operants that are subject to reinforcement by the attention of others. In this regard the somatizing patient's family environment can provide crucial contingencies of reinforcement for symptoms. The solicitude of family members may positively reinforce illness behavior. The patient's distress may provide a focus that distracts couples from problems in their relationship. For a healthy spouse (or other loved one) there are payoffs that come from caregiving, such as a sense of purpose and increased power or worth in the relationship.

Involvement of a significant other (typically a spouse or domestic partner) is an important component of our treatment. The significant other's involvement gives us access to another source of data about the patient's functioning, over and above the patient's self-report and the observations of the therapist. The benefit of additional data, of another window into the patient's world, itself would be sufficient grounds for sessions including the significant other, given how dependent mental health professionals are upon the narratives of their patients. But in addition to providing another perspective, the significant other also can provide therapeutic leverage. The significant other can be enlisted to modify the family environment to reduce pathogenic stress. The presence of a significant other who is cognizant of therapeutic goals and "on the same page" as the therapist is a great advantage compared with having the patient reside with a significant other who is either uninformed or perhaps at cross-purposes with the program of therapy. The involvement of a spouse or domestic partner in CBT is not the rule, but is very common across a range of clinical problems, including obesity (Black, Gleser, & Kooyers, 1990), chronic pain (Keefe et al., 1996), depression (Beach, Fincham, & Katz, 1998), and alcoholism (McCrady, Stout, Noel, Abrams, & Nelson, 1991; Rotunda & O'Farrell, 1997). With some exceptions, the involvement of a significant other in treatment has been found to be an effective option in the application of CBT. Our own experience and the feedback we have received from patients suggests that conjoint sessions attended by somatizers and their significant others are therapeutically very valuable.

Other behavior engaged in by somatizers can be viewed through the prism of operant conditioning. If frequent healthcare visits by somatizing patients serve to alleviate worry about health, albeit transiently, then medical help-seeking behavior is likely negatively reinforced through the reduction of anxiety and distress. Healthcare professionals' concern for and attentiveness to patients may positively reinforce the seeking of healthcare and facilitate the overuse of healthcare services. So, too, the avoidance of many normal activities and obligations, such as absenteeism from employment, can be regarded as an operant subject to reinforcement by the environment.

Investigation of the kind of "illness behavior" engaged in by somatizers and other medical patients has become a field in its own right. The next section will discuss an analytical framework derived from sociology in which some patient behavior is viewed as a kind of enactment or social role.

THE SICK ROLE

Role theory (Biddle, 1986) is a perspective within the social sciences from which, as Shakespeare (*As You Like It*, Act II, Scene 7) inimitably put it:

> All the world's a stage,
> And all the men and women merely players:
> They have their exits and their entrances;
> And one man in his time plays many parts.

Role theory regards each individual's actions as occurring within a collection of "parts" or roles. Roles are coherent patterns of behavior that are governed by the normative expectations of social groups and are inculcated through socialization, through rewards and punishments, and by the observation of role models. Thus we learn the behavior that is appropriate to being a teacher, doctor, mother, son, baseball player, political radical, macho guy, or "new woman." The language of the drama notwithstanding, in our roles we are not simply play-acting. Rather, we often so identify with our roles that they become the basic constituents of who we are and who we believe ourselves to be.

Sociologist Talcott Parsons was the first person to apply the ideas of role theory and the "dramaturgical" theory of social behavior to the study of illness. Parsons believed that both healers and patients could be seen as actors in a drama in which both had prescribed parts. The "sick role," as described by Parsons (1975), comprises interrelated kinds of requirements and exemptions. The sick person is not considered responsible for being in the grip of an illness, the amelioration of which also is deemed to be beyond the patient's control. Capacities to perform a variety of everyday roles are viewed as impaired, and the sick person is relieved of some obligations to function normally. In exchange for exoneration from various forms of responsibility, the patient is expected to accept the "illness" label and to cooperate with treatment by authorized healers. A related concept is a "patient identity" (Gara, Rosenberg, & Woolfolk, 1993), which refers to a perception of oneself as a medical patient that is central to one's sense of self. Despite much increased acceptance of mental disorders as legitimate forms of disability, the stigma attached to psychological problems of living continues to ensure that the most acceptable sick role involves having somatic versus psychological dysfunctions and displaying illness behavior that is related to physical symptoms.

Role theory suggests that eventually we become the roles that we play, provided that we play a role often, that the role is incentivized, and that contrary roles are disincentivized. From this perspective, somatizers who occupy the sick role in the absence of demonstrable somatic pathology are not malingerers. Those who chronically inhabit the sick role grow more disabled over time, and their impairment is genuine. Low expectations of self, much time spent focused on symptoms, social reinforcement of incapacity, and withdrawal from an active, productive life, all ultimately erode the capacity for normal functioning and produce authentic impairment. Frequent, chronic medical testing and treatment also may ingrain the sick role in patients.

In the case of somatization, the patient may become ensnared in various self-perpetuating vicious circles. Illness behavior can be reinforced in many ways and by many people. As the concept of secondary gain (Barsky & Klerman, 1983) attests, there are many rewards and exemptions attached to illness. As the sick role associated with somatization is "enacted," it may become entrenched via a variety of mechanisms. For some somatizers and hypochondriacs the very posing of the question "How do I know that I am not seriously ill?" introduces doubts, fears, and an obsessive focus that cannot be relinquished. In other cases the drama or melodrama of suffering and being cared for may, in some ways, have an appeal that a healthier life does not. Some somatizers come from families in which it was normal for someone to be sick. Illness "scripts" learned in childhood may emerge upon the occurrence of an aversive symptom. Sickness can function as a role to which the patient becomes attached, and the patient identity can be a "social station" that, despite its many disadvantages and discontents, feels fitting, normal, and, in some overall sense, comfortable to the patient (Mechanic, 1962).

Most investigators who have examined the link between somatization and possible benefits of illness behavior have concluded that somatization is associated with secondary gain (Gatchel, 2004; Rainville, Sobel, Hartigan, & Wright, 1997). Fishbain (1994, 1998) provides an instructive critical analysis of the construct of secondary gain and its relations to somatization, illness behavior, and the sick role. He identifies numerous "payoffs" that may motivate the sick role and constitute secondary gains of abnormal illness behavior:

1. Avoidance of an unpleasant or unsatisfactory life role or activity
2. Solicitude, sympathy, and concern from family and friends
3. Importance or power within the family
4. Avoidance of sex
5. Procuring drugs
6. Financial awards associated with disability
7. Retaining the spouse in a marriage
8. Avoidance of blame for one's failures or shortcomings
9. Punishment of others or revenge
10. Gratification of preexisting unresolved dependent strivings
11. Achieving justice or one's "just deserts"

For the most part, the elements of the sick role and its associated illness behavior and secondary gain that are features of somatization are not entirely within the patient's awareness or volition. Patients cannot "will" changes in their symptoms nor do they inevitably give up or suspend the sick role when contingencies change. For example, resolutions of symptom-related litigation or insurance claims do not invariably resolve perceived dysfunction or disability (Evans, 1992). Indeed, treatment can be successful even when litigation remains unresolved (Schofferman & Wasserman, 1994). Through interventions into the structure of the patient's life, as well as through influencing the patient's attitudes, beliefs, and conduct, inappropriate illness behavior can be disincentivized and salutary alternatives can be incentivized. Sometimes it is the patient's relationship with the healthcare system that must be a target of interventions (Smith et al., 1986b). In other cases, the patient's place in his or her family or workplace must be addressed. Our approach to secondary gain is to diminish it on all practicable fronts, while realizing that secondary gain and sick role considerations, though important, are but one set of factors that may serve to maintain somatization symptoms.

RATIONALE FOR AFFECTIVE COGNITIVE-BEHAVIORAL THERAPY

A biopsychosocial conceptualization of somatization is consonant with a broadly inclusive approach to assessment and treatment. In our own case it has led to a multifaceted psychosocial treatment approach that includes cognitive, experiential, interpersonal, and behavioral interventions. Our model of somatization emphasizes the interaction of physiology, cognition, emotion, behavior, and environment. We refer the reader back to the case of Rahim, introduced at the beginning of this chapter. Even before conducting a comprehensive assessment, we might make some tentative hypotheses about psychosocial factors contributing to his somatic symptoms, aside from possible organic factors. First, the occurrence and timing of his symptoms suggest that they may be stress-related. Rahim's cognitions related to his occupational, financial, and family contexts would be assessed in our case conceptualization. Second, Rahim's denial of negative affect in the face of such stressors is a diagnostic "red flag," a characteristic that we find frequently with somatizers. With somatizing patients who are in difficult circumstances, but who experience little negative affect, we spend much time attempting to elicit and identify affect. Additional areas of inquiry that would inform our conceptualization include the possibility of secondary gain. Do Rahim's symptoms provide any negative reinforcement, for example, allowing him to avoid work responsibilities or thoughts about his job, career, finances, or self-worth? Does the sick role free Rahim from any of his or his family's expectations for his success? Discussions with Rahim about these issues would provide the starting point of the assessment, case conceptualization, and treatment.

Our treatment for somatization disorder has evolved from a highly structured, 10-session manual-based individual CBT to a longer and more comprehensive treatment. The briefer intervention taught patients relaxation techniques to reduce stress, behavioral activation and communication skills to minimize the sick role, some minimal training in emotional awareness, and cognitive restructuring to alter and reduce dysfunctional cognitions. Given the complexities of cases we see, like Rahim's, an expansion of the treatment was warranted. Our current, expanded treatment not only provides more thorough CBT, but also emphasizes emotional awareness and acceptance in patients. Also, we have developed a more systematic intervention addressing the sick role, one that includes a highly systematic analysis of the functional significance of the sick role for the patient with somatization, the reinforcement contingencies consequating illness behavior, and the interpersonal relationships and life structures that provide the contexts for the sick role's enactment. This latter emphasis on and foregrounding of patients' relationships and living environment is nothing new. It can be found in approaches to therapy as diverse as family systems therapy, interpersonal therapy (IPT), and operant conditioning approaches.

Much of what we do with patients that goes beyond standard CBT has long been a staple of humanistic and psychoanalytic therapies and is coming to be emphasized by newer approaches that have grown out of the cognitive-behavioral tradition. Traditional cognitive approaches were based on a cognitive-appraisal theory of emotion (Arnold, 1960; Lazarus, 1966) in which dysfunctional cognitions were thought to generate aversive affects. Although this view was modified to be more *bi*directional and causally reciprocal by Teasdale (1983), much CBT has been directed to the reduction of aversive affect, largely through the modification of cognition that was assumed to be the source. Some approaches that have developed within the CBT framework have begun to change this emphasis on active control of emotion. Recent clinical work by such investigators as Linehan (1993), Hayes, Strosahl, and Wilson (1999), and Newman, Castonguay, Borkovec, and Molnar (2004) has placed emphasis on experiencing, tolerating, and accepting unpleasant emotion, rather than seeking its elimination. Recent formulations of generalized anxiety disorder (GAD) suggest that the function of this disorder's primary symptom (i.e., worry) may be to avoid, control, or attenuate emotional experience (Mennin, Heimberg, Turk, & Fresco, 2002; Roemer & Orsillo, 2002). The authors of these recent formulations of GAD also advocate experiential and acceptance approaches as a means of reducing worry. Samoilov and Goldfried's (2000) critique of standard CBT approaches suggests more emphasis on the elicitation of affect in therapy sessions may produce more effective treatment. The arguments of the revisionist theorists cited above frequently draw from basic work in cognitive neuroscience, work that suggests there are complex, manifold, and partially independent levels of cognitive and affective storage and processing (Izard, 1993; LeDoux, 1995). These "experiential" cognitive-behavioral treatments combine training aimed at either emotional exploration or emotional regulation. In an analysis of the perennial tensions between these two valid goals of therapy, Westen (2000) has cogently described the manifold and difficult therapeutic dilemmas regarding when and under what circumstances psychotherapists should attempt to assist patients in accessing and exploring affective states or, alternatively, in eliminating or attenuating those states. He argues that traditional CBT approaches have erred in the direction of attempts to control emotions and failed to address adequately the implicit, tacit, nonverbal, and emotional aspects of existence. Our work with patients with somatization is predicated on the assumption that the palpable impact of CBT on somatization is not only enhanced by the kinds of modifications in CBT that we and others have endorsed, but that the potential of the approach can only be fully realized within the context of a method that places more emphasis on emotional processing.

In the chapters that follow, we make more systematic and explicit an aspect of our treatment that has been insufficiently emphasized in previous formulations and presentations (Allen, Woolfolk, & Gara, 2001; Allen, Woolfolk, Lehrer, Gara, & Escobar, 2001) of our work: its emphasis on emotional exploration, differentiation, expression, and acceptance.

CHAPTER 4

Assessment

Despite the prevalence and cost of somatization syndromes, they often go unrecognized in both psychiatric and medical practices (Fabrega et al., 1988; Fink et al., 1999; Peveler et al., 1997). Patients are likely to mention only the complaints that they consider relevant to a given practitioner, even though they (patients) may be aware of other distressing physical and/or emotional symptoms. Often mental health professionals and their patients focus their attention on emotional, cognitive, behavioral, and environmental issues while curtailing discussions of somatic complaints. Lacking extensive training in somatic illness, nonmedical mental health providers may feel incapable of assessing or evaluating physical symptomatology. Instead, these practitioners may encourage patients to seek further medical evaluation of their physical symptoms by physicians without examining the larger biopsychosocial context in which the symptoms occur. In this way, mental health clinicians inadvertently may encourage unnecessary medical testing that reinforces dysfunctional illness behavior and beliefs. Before referring patients for piecemeal medical testing, a clinician should look at the overall pattern of physical symptomatology and assess for the presence of somatization.

> Lauren was a 33-year-old woman seeking psychotherapy for a long history of depressed and anxious moods that she attributed to being a child of an alcoholic parent. In addition to her emotional difficulties, she reported disabling fatigue that had been diagnosed as chronic fatigue syndrome. Over the course of therapy, Lauren complained of numerous, recurrent physical symptoms that she and her therapist, a doctoral-level

psychologist, regarded as "medical symptoms" to be addressed by a medical practitioner. The therapist never incorporated those symptoms into the case conceptualization or treatment. Instead, attempting to ensure the patient received comprehensive treatment, the therapist avoided discussions of Lauren's physical symptoms and, on multiple occasions, referred the patient for medical evaluations. By the time Lauren reached our clinic, her primary care physician had begun to suspect somatization and had arrived at a preliminary diagnosis of somatization disorder. This diagnosis was confirmed during the extensive testing that is part of our research protocol and will be described later in this chapter.

We, of course, would not suggest that clinicians assume all physical symptoms are related to psychopathology. We simply want to encourage mental health clinicians to communicate with patients' medical practitioners to access all information relevant to a biopsychosocial formulation of the case. When unexplained medical symptoms are multiple and of long duration, the possible presence of a somatoform disorder should at least be explored and perhaps ruled out. In a patient who turns out to have an underlying somatoform disorder, neglecting the biological, psychological, behavioral, or environmental factors may not only result in a failure to alleviate, but also aggravate the problem. Medical practitioners, trained to identify and treat organic disease underlying presenting symptoms, also can err in focusing on the aspects of their specialty isolated from a comprehensive biopsychosocial context. Missing an aspect of these complex, mind–body cases may set the stage for extensive diagnostic excursions in search of uncommon physical diseases. Unnecessary diagnostic procedures, hospitalizations, and surgeries are expensive, disruptive, and potentially detrimental to patients' physical and psychological well-being. Excessive medical procedures may create iatrogenic illness in patients. Equally problematic is the message communicated: that any distressing physical symptom is a sign of disease, a dysfunctional belief frequently held by somatoform disorder patients. To avoid such unproductive and potentially destructive activities, healthcare providers have been urged to assess for somatoform disorders (Barksy & Borus, 1995; Katon, Sullivan, & Walker, 2001).

In this chapter, we describe methods for identifying and diagnosing somatization. We also discuss the use of assessment in informing and enhancing treatment as well as in evaluating the effect of treatment. Ideally, assessment not only provides the requisite information for differential diagnosis, case conceptualization, and treatment planning, but also can enhance the therapeutic relationship. Because of the complexity of many somatization cases, we encourage clinicians to think of assessment as a process that occurs throughout treatment. Over the course of treatment, as patients become more comfortable, they may begin to disclose more information. Many somatization patients have complex symptom histories that they may not fully recall on a single assessment occasion. It has been our experience that as therapy unfolds the therapeutic work itself may cue various recollections of symptoms and circumstances that may have precipitated symptoms. Initial diagnoses and hypothesized contributing factors should be reconsidered as the case develops.

To illustrate our approach to assessment, we presented the case of Lauren and will present the case of Manuel. The two cases are described because they are representative of the two most common presentations: (1) an emotionally distressed psychotherapy patient (Lauren) with somatization symptoms and (2) a medical patient (Manuel) whose medical practitioner has decided that psychotherapy, rather than or in addition to biomedical intervention, is most likely to ease physical complaints.

Manuel was not certain what was happening to him. As he sat down to eat dinner one night, he felt an intense pain in his chest. He was frightened and somewhat disoriented. Immediately, Manuel began to think that he might be having a heart attack. "What's wrong?" his wife Carmen asked. "I think I need to go to the hospital," Manuel replied. Several hours later, Manuel and Carmen left the hospital reassured that he had not experienced a coronary. A referral to a cardiologist resulted in a thallium stress test. The results of this test suggested that Manuel might have a blockage in one of his coronary arteries. He was scheduled for an angiogram, a procedure that required general anesthesia and a day away from work. As his cardiologist put it, "We went into the artery, looked at it, and it is clean. There is no occlusion of the artery. The thallium stress test gave us a false positive." Three weeks after his scare at the dinner table, many hours of interaction with healthcare workers and thousands of dollars in medical expenses later, Manuel's heart had received a clean bill of health.

What had not emerged during the crisis following the acute episode was that Manuel had been experiencing unexplained medical symptoms for many years. He had chronic "stress" headaches, pain in his jaw, a "sensitive stomach," and various other gastrointestinal symptoms, and numbness in his extremities. But no healthcare provider had ever comprehended the larger pattern of somatization. Had Manuel been examined via a semistructured clinical interview, such as the Structured Clinical Interview for DSM-IV Disorders (SCID), he would have qualified, by a considerable margin, for a diagnosis of somatization disorder. The SCID would have also ruled out panic disorder, a disorder often implicated in cases when individuals falsely believe they are having heart attacks. Manuel's pain at the dinner table had been real, but the pain was not from a malfunction of his circulatory system. His pain was one symptom in a pattern of somatization symptomatology, a pattern that had gone undetected and undiagnosed for many years.

When asking patients with somatization about their presenting problems, it is important to ascertain information about how they were referred to therapy and their thoughts and feelings about the referral. Each patient has a unique story, though there are common themes. Frustration, helplessness, and uncertainty almost always are part of what must be discussed. Unexplained symptoms with uncertain prospects of remedy almost always induce frustration, if not intense distress. The assessment and treatment of somatization is among the most inexact of endeavors, with uncertain implications. This uncertainty must be acknowledged, but the possibility of tangible therapeutic assistance also must be asserted and advanced as the reason for an exploration of symptoms.

CLINICAL INTERVIEW

When a patient like Manuel presents for psychotherapy (or the somatization component of cases like Lauren's is revealed), the first priority is to clarify the presenting problem(s) and related medical pathology and psychopathology. We recommend a thorough review of medical and psychiatric history as well as a discussion of current occupational, social, and physical functioning. Whenever possible, such information is requested not only from patients themselves, but also from their physicians and family members.

A diagnosis of DSM-IV somatization disorder (or of moderate levels of somatization) requires clinicians to review patients' lifetime history of 33 different physical symptoms and to determine the status of those symptoms, a time-consuming and complex task. Because most clinicians make diagnostic decisions based on unstructured patient interviews, many symptoms experienced by somatizers may never be discussed. Histories of somatization symptoms and abnormal illness behavior may be obscured by patients' narratives of their lives.

More accurate diagnoses may be achieved using a structured interview schedule, such as the SCID (First, Spitzer, Gibbon, & Williams, 1997), and a medical history review. The SCID provides questions to guide the clinician through the diagnostic criteria for the somatoform

disorders (somatization disorder, hypochondriasis, undifferentiated somatoform disorder, pain disorder, and body dysmorphic disorder) as
well as the other major psychiatric disorders. The somatization disorder
section of the SCID requires the clinician ask in detail about the patient's
lifetime experience with each physical symptom. The impact of each
symptom experienced on the patient's behavior is explored. Also, patients are asked for any previous medical diagnoses and medical recommendations for each symptom. Because patients' responses to questions about the organic basis of symptoms are not necessarily reliable,
patients' physicians are consulted. Only medically unexplained symptoms are counted toward the somatization diagnosis.

Although the somatization section of the SCID may seem tedious
to the clinician, we have found very few somatization patients respond
negatively to its administration. In fact, most seem to appreciate the
interviewer's careful attention to their somatic symptomatology. We
have come to view the somatization disorder section of the SCID as a
means of jumpstarting the therapeutic alliance for patients like Manuel
and as a means of deepening the patient–clinician bond for patients
like Lauren. For many somatization patients, this interview is the first
time a healthcare practitioner has extensively evaluated each of their
symptoms.

In addition to enhancing the patient–clinician relationship, the
SCID, medical history review, and physician consultation can facilitate
differential diagnosis. General medical conditions, such as rheumatoid
arthritis, inflammatory bowel disease, and so on, may be excluded.
The interviewer can distinguish between hypochondriasis and somatization by clarifying whether the distress is caused more by the
patient's interpretations of symptoms (for example, that the recurrence
of the symptoms suggests a fatal illness) or by the symptoms themselves. Also, because the SCID requires the clinician inquire into the
patient's lifetime experience with other psychiatric disorders (affective,
anxiety, psychotic, and substance dependence disorders), other psychiatric explanations for symptoms can be excluded. Of course, the presentation of a general medical condition or a nonsomatoform psychiatric illness does not exclude the possibility of a comorbid somatoform
disorder. In fact, these comorbid conditions are present in some of the
most complex cases.

In the case of Manuel, the administration of the SCID, review of his
medical history, and consultation with his primary physician revealed a
long history of pain complaints (i.e., chest pain, headaches, jaw pain)
without any associated diagnosed organic pathology. Our assessment
also uncovered a prior diagnosis of irritable bowel syndrome (IBS),

whose symptoms seemed to wax and wane. Although not as disabling as his other symptoms, his abdominal pain, bloating, and diarrhea were distressing. Manuel had received no other medical diagnoses over the course of his life. Additional unexplained and disturbing symptoms he had experienced intermittently were numbness in his extremities and erectile dysfunction. Taken together, Manuel's symptoms met DSM-IV criteria for somatization disorder, an unlikely diagnosis to be considered had the SCID not been administered, perhaps because the patient never volunteered complaints about his gastrointestinal system or sexual functioning. The remaining sections of the SCID revealed some anxiety symptoms that were insufficient for an anxiety disorder diagnosis.

In addition to providing information with which to make a preliminary diagnosis, the assessment interviews provide the foundation of the case conceptualization. We supplement the medical history review and SCID with a deeper exploration of the symptoms: What has been the course of the symptoms? What were the coinciding life events, if any? What treatments were received for the symptoms? How have significant others responded to the symptoms? What thoughts and feelings does the patient have about the symptoms? Input from family members can shed light on the symptoms, the patient's experience with symptoms, and related events.

How Much Medical Assessment Is Enough?

Nonmedical mental health practitioners, lacking the background to determine organic basis of symptoms, are likely to feel uneasy discouraging additional medical procedures for physical symptoms. We have handled this dilemma by recommending patients' primary physicians follow Smith and colleagues' (1986b) treatment suggestions for somatization patients (described in Chapter 2). That is, patients should be seen regularly (i.e., every 4–6 weeks) by their primary care physicians. Physicians will conduct physical examinations at these visits without prescribing unnecessary diagnostic procedures, surgical interventions, or hospitalizations. Therapists contact primary physicians for updates on patients' medical status.

We incorporate "likely somatization" symptoms into the case conceptualization when the aforementioned clinical interview suggests any of the following:

- A patient reports a lifetime history of multiple physical symptoms with unclear or no diagnoses.
- A patient reports seeing many doctors and receiving many diag-

nostic procedures with inconsistent findings for more than one symptom.

- A patient reports a pattern of physicians, family members, and/ or friends being "unable to understand" or "fed up" with the patient's physical symptoms.
- Symptoms are described graphically or dramatically. For example, a patient may state that he or she "screams" in pain or that the pain was a 100 on a scale from 0 to 10.
- There is strong evidence of secondary gain associated with the symptoms.

SELF-REPORT QUESTIONNAIRES

In our clinical work with somatization patients, we use only two self-report indices: (1) the Severity of Somatic Symptoms Scale to assess the progress of treatment, and (2) symptom monitoring forms (i.e., diaries) to identify situations, thoughts, and emotions related to the somatic symptomatology. At the initial evaluation session, we ask patients to complete the Severity of Somatic Symptoms Scale (Appendix C), which asks patients to rate the severity of each of 40 somatic symptoms over the previous month. In an effort to avoid encouraging excessive focus on physical symptoms, we readminister the Severity of Somatic Symptoms Scale every 4 weeks, instead of every week, to assess change in treatment. Patients whose functioning is moderately to severely impaired by their physical symptoms tend to score over 40 on the Severity of Somatic Symptoms Scale. In clinical practice we are interested in a patient's score on this scale relative to his or her previous score. We have found a 25% reduction in the Severity of Somatic Symptoms Scale total score to be an indication of clinically meaningful change.

Because our use of symptom diaries is such an integral part of our therapy, we describe their use in Chapters 6–9.

ASSESSMENT IN RESEARCH SETTINGS

Structured Clinical Interviews

The interview schedules most often used by researchers to assess somatoform disorders are the SCID, the Composite International Diagnostic Interview (CIDI; World Health Organization, 1994a), and the CIDI's predecessor, the Diagnostic Interview Schedule (DIS; Robins, Helzer, Croughan, & Ratcliff, 1981). Both the SCID and the CIDI provide questions to guide an interviewer through the diagnostic criteria for the major psychiatric disorders. The CIDI, comprising a completely standardized set of close-ended questions, to be answered yes or no, can be administered by a trained layperson interviewer. A diagnosis is generated without clinical interpretation, based entirely on symptom occurrence patterns. The semistructured SCID includes questions to be posed verbatim and authorizes a set of follow-up probes that can be modified, based on the respondent's answers and the interviewer's clinical judgment, to ensure diagnostic criteria are met. Many follow-up questions are open-ended to encourage patients to describe symptoms in their own words. These more open-ended discussions allow interviewers to clarify the meaning of patients' responses to the more structured questions. The knowledge base and clinical experience of a trained clinician, as opposed to that of a layperson, are necessary to conduct the SCID. Another difference between the CIDI and the SCID is that SCID interviewers are encouraged to base their diagnostic decisions not only on the respondent's answers to interview questions and the clinician's observations during the interview, but also on information from other sources (such as physicians and family members). In addition to differences in modes of administration, the somatoform sections of the CIDI and the SCID differ in content. Whereas the SCID covers DSM-IV diagnoses, the CIDI covers DSM-IV and ICD-10 diagnoses.

Two other interview schedules for assessing somatoform disorders are the Schedules for Clinical Assessment in Neuropsychiatry (SCAN; World Health Organization, 1994b) and the Somatoform Disorders Schedule (SDS; World Health Organization, 1994c). The SCAN is a semistructured interview for diagnosing the principal DSM-IV and ICD-10 disorders. Like the SCID, the SCAN allows the interviewer some flexibility in probing symptomatology and in requesting supplemental information from third parties. The SDS reviews only DSM-IV and ICD-10 somatoform disorders, instead of all major psychiatric disorders. The SDS follows the fully structured format of the CIDI so that it can be administered by a layperson with minimal training.

No consensus has been reached as to the best interview schedule. Although the CIDI, SCID, and SCAN are used widely in research, little effort has been directed toward examining the psychometric properties of their somatoform sections. Some investigators claim the validity of semistructured interviews, such as the SCID and SCAN, is superior to that of the fully structured CIDI and SDS interviews (Spitzer, 1983). First, a greater volume of accurate information may be elicited by interviewers who use clinical judgment in their questions and ratings of responses in a format that allows for some latitude in exploring patients' symptoms. Second, semistructured interviews allow the interviewer access to information from third parties. This second point is critical in assessing somatization symptoms. For various reasons, including patients' defensiveness and poor physician–patient communication, few patients ever state directly that a given symptom is medically unexplained. By relying upon interviewees' descriptions of the nature of their physical symptoms, the CIDI and SDS may result in fewer somatoform disorder diagnoses than do the SCID and SCAN. On the other hand, some investigators suggest the flexibility allowed by the SCID and SCAN may come at a cost to reliability. Clinical judgment allows for variability across interviews. All of the somatoform sections of these interviews ultimately may prove to be reliable and valid. Thus far, only the CIDI has published data demonstrating its reliability (Semler et al., 1987; Wittchen, 1994).

We recommend that the selection of a diagnostic instrument be based upon intended purpose. If the primary goal is accuracy of diagnosis, we recommend using the SCID or SCAN administered by well-trained clinician-interviewers who consult relevant medical records or physicians. Epidemiological researchers, interested in assessing very large numbers of respondents, often use fully structured interviews, such as the CIDI or SDS, that can be administered by trained laypeople and are less costly in terms of time and money.

Screening Instruments

Attempting to reduce the time and energy required to make a definitive diagnosis of somatization disorder, a number of researchers have developed brief measures to identify patients who are likely to have multiple unexplained physical symptoms. The standard approach to screening for somatization disorders involves the use of self-report questionnaires asking respondents about their experience with multiple physical symptoms. Although many somatically focused questionnaires have been administered as screens, three instruments were specifically designed for such purposes. Two measures were developed 20 years ago to identify patients likely to meet criteria for DSM-III somatization disorder (Othmer & DeSouza, 1985; Swartz, Hughes, et al., 1986). A third measure that aims to identify not only the most severe, but also moderately severe cases of somatization is the World Health Organization's (1994c) Screener for Somatoform Disorders (SSD), which screens for ICD-10 somatoform disorders. All three of these screening questionnaires ask respondents to indicate which of a predefined list of physical symptoms they have experienced during a specified time frame. As illustrated in Table 4.1, the three screening questionnaires assess relatively few of the same symptoms.

The use of these three screening tools has costs and benefits. Their advantages include brevity and ease of administration and scoring. Each can be completed and scored in about 5 minutes. Furthermore, some research supports the efficacy of these measures in identifying somatization or somatization disorder (Bucholz, Dinwiddie, Reich, Shayka, & Cloninger, 1993; Garcia-Campayo, Sanz-Carrillo, Perez-Echeverria, Campos, & Lobo, 1996; Kroenke, Spitzer, deGruy, & Swindle, 1998; Othmer & DeSouza, 1985; Smith & Brown, 1990; Swartz, Hughes, et al., 1986). Nevertheless, the scales have significant shortcomings. Most problematic is each scale's inability to distinguish between medically explained and medically unexplained symptoms.

TABLE 4.1. Overview of Somatization Screening Questionnaires

	SSD	Swartz, Hughes, et al. (1986)	Othmer & DeSouza (1985)
Time frame of symptoms	6 months	Lifetime	Lifetime
Number of possible symptoms	12	11	7
Number of required symptoms	3	5	3
Extremity pain	*	*	*
Abdominal pain	*	*	
Dizziness	*	*	
Gas and/or bloating	*	*	
Fatigue	*		
Headaches	*		
Back pain	*		
Trouble sleeping	*		
Palpitations	*		
Numbness or tingling	*		
Lightheadedness	*		
Dry mouth	*		
Nausea		*	
Chest pain		*	
Fainting		*	
Diarrhea		*	
Weakness		*	
Feeling sickly		*	
Vomiting		*	*
Shortness of breath			*
Menstrual problems			*
Sexual pain/problems			*
Lump in throat			*
Amnesia			*

Note. SSD, Screener for Somatoform Disorders (World Health Organization, 1994c); * indicates symptom is included in screening questionnaire.

Consequently, the somatization scores of medically ill patients are spuriously inflated. Other shortcomings have been associated with each scale. The tests developed by Othmer and DeSouza (1985) and Swartz, Hughes, and colleagues (1986) to identify full somatization disorder may fail to detect moderate somatization (Kroenke et al., 1998). To our knowledge, the psychometric properties of the SSD have not yet been published.

More recently, screening instruments have been designed to assess only those physical symptoms that are medically unexplained. The Screening for Somatoform Symptoms (SOMS; Rief, Hiller, Geissner, & Fichter, 1995; Rief, Hiller, & Heuser, 1997) is a self-report questionnaire listing 53 symptoms from the somatoform sections of DSM-IV and ICD-10. The SOMS instructions state that respondents should indicate which symptoms they experienced within the last 2 years "for which no clear causes have been found by a physician and which have affected your subjective well-being." Symptoms that respondents believe to be organically based are not rated. Research on the SOMS's psychometric properties suggests it may be effective and efficient for identifying current levels of somatization (Rief et al., 1995, 1997).

Taking a slightly different approach to teasing apart medically explained and medically unexplained symptoms with a self-report inventory, our research team developed the Somatic Symptom Questionnaire (SSQ; Woolfolk, Allen, Gara, & Escobar, 1998). Respondents to the SSQ indicate whether they have *ever* experienced each of 40 symptoms from the somatization sections of the CIDI and SCID. For symptoms experienced, patients indicate (1) if the symptom was explained by a physical illness or an accident, (2) if the symptom prompted the seeking of medical attention, and (3) the diagnostic explanation for the symptom (see Appendix D). Symptoms that both prompted the seeking of treatment and were not explained by a physical illness or accident are counted toward a total somatization score. Although preliminary, the psychometric properties of the SSQ suggest it may be a reliable and valid tool for identifying somatization disorder (Woolfolk et al., 1998).

The SOMS and the less well-established SSQ may provide expedient alternatives for detecting somatization disorders. The SOMS and SSQ provide comprehensive symptom counts only for respondent-reported medically unexplained symptoms. Though approximating the content of fully structured clinical interviews, the SOMS and SSQ are substantially briefer and simpler to administer than structured clinical interviews. The disadvantage of the SOMS and SSQ is their reliance on patients' reports of explanations for their symptoms. Just as with fully structured clinical interviews, somatization symptoms may be underreported on the SOMS and SSQ. In all, we believe both the SOMS and SSQ possess a combination of brevity and comprehensiveness that makes them the most promising screening instruments for somatization. Despite their utility, the gold standard for making somatoform diagnoses remains the structured clinical interview.

Severity of Somatization

Although valuable in the diagnosis of somatization, the structured clinical interviews described above do not assess the severity of somatization symptoms. In effect, each symptom is given equal weight and is used to generate a categorical decision regarding diagnosis. The somatization disorder diagnosis is based on the occurrence of somatization symptoms over the course of one's entire life. Therefore, diagnostic interviews, assessing the presence or absence of somatization symptoms over an individual's lifetime, are structurally incapable of detecting changes in somatization disorder. Even if successfully treated patients experience dramatic improvement in their unexplained physical symptoms, their diagnostic status will not change (assuming patients give accurate accounts of their lifetime experience with somatization symptoms).

Various methods have been employed to assess the severity of somatization. Table 4.2 lists the scales of somatic symptom severity that have been used to examine the severity of somatization.

The Symptom Checklist—Revised (SCL-90-R; Derogatis, 1983) is a 90-item multidimensional inventory assessing psychopathology with nine subscales: somatization, obsession–compulsion, interpersonal sensitivity, depression, anxiety, hostility, phobic anxiety, paranoid ideation, and psychoticism. These subscales were originally de-

TABLE 4.2. Measures of Severity of Somatization

Measure	Number of symptoms	Time frame	Rating scale
SCL-90-R (Derogatis, 1983)	12	1 week	5-point scale
PHQ-15 (Kroenke, Spitzer, & Williams, 2002)	15	4 weeks	3-point scale
Severity of Somatic Symptoms Scale (SSS; Allen, Woolfolk, Lehrer, et al., 2001)	36 for men 40 for women	1 month	8-point scale
SOMS-7 (Rief & Hiller, 2003)	48 for men 52 for women	1 week	5-point scale

rived from factor analyses (Derogatis, 1983). Respondents use 5-point Likert-type items to rate how bothersome each symptom has been over the previous week. The 12-item somatization subscale of commonly experienced physical symptoms has been used as a stand-alone measure of somatization severity (Katon et al., 1991; McLeod, Budd, & McClelland, 1997) and appears sensitive to change (McLeod et al., 1997). Despite the somatization subscale's popularity, some researchers have discouraged the use of the SCL-90-R's individual subscales as a means of assessing distinct domains of psychopathology. It seems the scale's original 9-factor structure has not been replicated and the subscales appear to be highly intercorrelated (Cyr, McKenna-Foley, & Peacock, 1985; Hardt, Gerbershagen, & Franke, 2000). Still, the total SCL-90-R score is considered a sound measure of overall distress. Severity on its somatization subscale may be a more valid indicator of overall emotional distress than of the severity of somatization disorder.

The Patient Health Questionnaire (PHQ-15; Kroenke, Spitzer, & Williams, 2002) has recently been promoted as a somatization severity scale. The PHQ-15 is the somatic symptom subscale of the PHQ, the self-report questionnaire designed to assess for psychiatric disorders in primary care (Spitzer et al., 1999). The PHQ-15 comprises 15 physical symptoms that are rated on 3-point Likert-type items (0 = not bothered at all, 1 = bothered a little, 2 = bothered a lot) to indicate how bothersome symptoms were during the past month. These 15 symptoms have been found to be among the most prevalent somatic symptoms presented in general medical practice (Kroenke, Arrington, & Mangelsdorff, 1990; Liu, Clark, & Eaton, 1997). Because the PHQ-15 is a relatively new instrument, less research has been conducted on it than on older measures. The one study examining its psychometric properties, in a sample of 6,000 general internal medicine, family practice, and obstetrics-gynecology patients, found it to have high reliability, conceived as internal consistency (Cronbach's alpha = 0.80), and to be associated with functional impairment and use of healthcare services (Kroenke et al., 2002). Its test–retest reliability, association with other measures of somatization symptoms, and sensitivity to changes in symptomatology have not yet been examined.

The Severity of Somatic Symptoms Scale (SSS; Allen, Woolfolk, Lehrer, et al., 2001) is made up of 40 symptoms selected from the somatization sections of the CIDI and SCID (see Appendix C). Each symptom is rated for severity on an 8-point Likert-type item. The SSS is a more comprehensive measure of somatization disorder severity than are the SCL-90-R and PHQ-15 somatization subscales, which assess a minority of the symptoms reported by patients with somatization disorder. As a measure of change, the wider net cast by the SSS may better capture the fluctuating nature of somatization symptoms than do less extensive measures. As is often the case with these patients, when one symptom remits it may simply be replaced by a new symptom, suggesting little change in the overall severity of somatization. In such instances, total scores on brief measures of somatization severity might change significantly, whereas the total SSS score is likely to indicate that little change in overall somatization severity has occurred. Findings from our laboratory indicate the SSS has high internal and test–retest reliability and is sensitive to symptomatic change (Allen, Woolfolk, Lehrer, et al., 2001).

Some researchers have used daily symptom diaries to assess severity of somatization (Allen, Woolfolk, & Gara, 2001; Greene & Blanchard, 1994; Van Dulmen et al., 1996). Daily symptom diaries not only have face validity, but also provide important information that is fine-grained, individualized, and standardized. These assessment virtues are crucial for a syndrome whose symptoms vary from day to day. Because diaries require severity ratings be made every day, they may more validly assess patients' symptomatology for a specified timeframe (e.g., 1 week, 1 month, etc.) than a questionnaire completed retrospectively at a single evaluation session. Past research on somatization syndromes has shown diaries to have acceptable psychometric properties. The literature on IBS demonstrates diary scores to be highly reliable and sensitive to change (Greene & Blanchard, 1994; Van Dulmen et al., 1996). Our own research on somatization disorder shows diaries have good test–retest reliability over a 2-week interval ($r = .86$) and are sensitive measures of symptomatic change (Allen, Woolfolk, & Gara, 2001). Critics of diaries question whether respondents actually record the data at the times and places the instructions require.

Unfortunately, none of the aforementioned severity questionnaires nor the daily symptom diaries specifically measure the severity only of physical symptoms that are medically unexplained. Like some of the somatization screening questionnaires, self-report severity scales are hampered by their inability to assess the status of patients' physical symptoms. Because these self-report questionnaires fail to distinguish between organic and functional symptoms, they may assess overall physical discomfort better than somatization severity.

Attempting to create a scale assessing the severity of only medically unexplained physical symptoms, Rief and Hiller modified their Screening for Somatoform Symptoms (SOMS) to include severity ratings for the past 7 days (SOMS-7; Rief & Hiller, 2003). The SOMS-7 requires patients to rate the amount of distress they experienced, on a 5-point Likert-type item, from each of a comprehensive list of somatization symptoms as defined by DSM-IV and ICD-10. Patients rate the severity of only those symptoms they consider to be medically unexplained. Just as with the SOMS, because respondents themselves make the distinction between medically explained and unexplained symptoms, the SOMS-7 may not be as accurate as clinician-administered measures. An initial study suggests the SOMS-7 has good internal consistency, test–retest reliability, and sensitivity to change (Rief & Hiller, 2003).

The best measure of somatization severity depends upon the aims of the assessment. The PHQ-15 can be completed most quickly. The SSS requires a few more minutes to complete than does the PHQ-15, but it covers a wider range of symptoms. The SOMS-7, though more time-consuming than the others, is the only severity scale to assess somatization, as opposed to somatic symptoms.

Use of Medical Services

As discussed in Chapter 2, the healthcare utilization practices of patients with multiple unexplained symptoms are a major public health concern. Many treatment studies with these patients target medical service utilization as a primary outcome measure (Creed et al., 2003; Hiller, Fichter, & Rief, 2003; Smith et al., 1995; Sumathipala et al., 2000). If a treatment reduces somatization in a clinically meaningful way, the intervention should be associated not only with reductions in discomfort, but also with reductions in medical treatment and healthcare costs. Investigators have taken different approaches to examining healthcare utilization. Some have asked patients to keep healthcare diaries in which each healthcare visit and procedure is recorded (Sumathipala et al., 2000). Patients' use of analgesics and other medication may be included in their healthcare diaries (Lidbeck, 1997). A more comprehensive approach to studying healthcare utilization involves collecting medical billing records from all healthcare providers and from all health insurance companies so that number, type, and cost of medical procedures can be documented (e.g., Hiller et al., 2003; Smith et al., 1995). Although conducting such elaborate assessment procedures is impractical in many settings, we encourage clinicians and researchers to inquire into their patients' healthcare utilization. Patient-recorded diaries of medical services and of medication consumption is a relatively efficient method for evaluating patients' illness behavior and healthcare utilization.

Functional Impairment

Given that somatization often affects various domains of functioning, we recommend that researchers and clinicians examine patients' behavioral limitations. Occupational, recreational, and social functioning as well as activities of daily living can all be assessed with questionnaires or with patient diaries.

The Medical Outcomes Study 36-Item Short Form Health Survey is a brief and comprehensive self-report questionnaire (MOS SF-36; Ware & Sherbourne, 1992). It comprises 36 items in the following eight subscales: physical functioning, social functioning, role functioning, mental health, vitality, bodily pain, general health perceptions, and change in health. Its items are scored variously on 2-point, 3-point, 5-point, or 6-point Likert-type items. Although some research has suggested that all the MOS SF-36 subscales are reliable and valid (Thumboo et al., 1999), the physical functioning subscale appears to be the most psychometrically sound (McHorney, Ware, Lu, & Sherbourne, 1994). The 10-item physical functioning subscale inquires into patients' ability to perform different activities of daily living (such as climbing one flight of stairs, walking more than a mile, or lifting or carrying groceries). Although the physical functioning subscale is sensitive to changes in impairment in patients meeting DSM-IV criteria for somatization disorder (Allen, Woolfolk, & Gara, 2001; Allen et al., 2006), it may not capture the physical limitations experienced by less severely disturbed somatizers, for whom the scale may have a psychometric measurement floor effect (McHorney et al., 1994). In 1996, a new version of the MOS SF-36, the SF-36v2 (Ware & Kosinski, 1996), was introduced in order to improve the psychometric properties of the overall scale and its subscales. The SF-36v2 includes revisions of some of the MOS-SF-36's subscales, though not of the physical functioning subscale.

The Sickness Impact Profile (SIP) is a 136-item measure divided into 12 subscales assessing a broad range of functioning, including physical, emotional, interpersonal, occupational, and leisure (Bergner, Bobbitt, Carter, & Gilson, 1981). A shorter version of the SIP, the SIP68 has also been developed and widely studied (de Bruin, Buys, de Witte, & Diederiks, 1994). Although both versions of the SIP have been shown to be reliable and valid measures of quality of life (de Bruin, Diederiks, de Witte, Stevens, & Philipsen, 1997), they have not been used as widely in the somatization literature as the MOS SF-36 has been. A limitation of the SIP is its length; even the abbreviated version of the SIP is substantially longer than the MOS SF-36 or SF-36v2.

Psychiatric Distress

Given the high rates of emotional distress associated with somatization, we encourage clinicians and researchers to assess for concomitant psychopathology, most often depression and/or anxiety. Three of the four structured diagnostic interviews described earlier in this chapter (CIDI, SCID, and SCAN) can be used to identify comorbid DSM-IV or ICD-10 psychiatric disorders. A widely used measure of severity of overall psychopathology is the SCL-90-R total score (Derogatis, 1983). Severity of depression and anxiety can be assessed with self-report or clinician-administered questionnaires. The Beck Depression Inventory (BDI; Beck, Ward, Mendelson, Mock, & Erbaugh, 1961), Center for Epidemiologic Studies Depression scale (CES-D; Radloff, 1977), and Zung Self-Rating Depression Scale (Zung, 1965) are well established and psychometrically sound self-report measures of depression. The State–Trait Anxiety Inventory (STAI; Spielberger, Gorsuch, & Lushene, 1970) and Beck Anxiety Inventory (BAI; Beck, Epstein, Brown, & Steer, 1988) are reliable and valid measures of anxiety. The most widely used clinician-administered measures of depression and anxiety are the Hamilton Rating Scales for Depression (Hamilton, 1960, 1967) and the Hamilton Rating Scale for Anxiety (Hamilton, 1959), respectively.

Associated Cognitive and Behavioral Disturbances

Recently, Rief, Hiller, and Margraf (1998) constructed a questionnaire designed to examine the cognitive disturbances associated with, and presumably exacerbating, somatoform disorders. The Cognitions about Body and Health Questionnaire (CABHQ; Rief, Hiller, & Margraf, 1998) consists of 31 statements, each of which is rated on a 4-point Likert-type scale. The questionnaire includes five subscales: catastrophizing interpretation of bodily complaints, autonomic sensations, bodily weakness, intolerance of bodily complaints, and health habits. The questionnaire's total scale appears to have high internal consistency (Cronbach's alpha ≥ 0.80) and to discriminate between somatoform and nonsomatoform patients (Rief, Hiller, & Margraf, 1998). All of the subscales, except health habits, also appear to discriminate between somatoform and nonsomatoform patients and to have adequate internal consistency, especially within clinical samples (Rief, Hiller, & Margraf, 1998). Researchers may be interested in using this measure to examine cognitive models of somatization.

The Somatic Symptom Amplification Scale (SSAS; Barsky et al., 1990) was designed to assess a "cognitive style" that has been ascribed to patients with hypochondriasis and, possibly, to all somatoform patients. Somatosensory amplification is the tendency to experience bodily sensations as intense, aversive, and/or distressing (Barsky et al., 1990). In theory, somatosensory amplification may play a causal role in these disorders. The SSAS questions respondents about their sensitivity to various mild physical sensations, such as hearing loud noises or bruising. The SSAS's 10 items are scored on 5-point Likert-type scales. Research indicates the instrument has good test–retest reliability and internal consistency and is highly correlated with hypochondriacal symptomatology (Barsky et al., 1990).

The Whiteley Index is a 14-item self-report questionnaire developed to assess for hypochondriacal attitudes (Pilowsky, 1967). Some researchers ask respondents to rate the 14 items on binary scales (Pilowsky, 1967; Speckens, Spinhoven, Sloekers, Bolk, & van Hemert, 1996), while others (Barsky et al., 1992) use 5-point Likert-type items (1 = not at all to 5 = a great deal). Although Pilowsky's data indicates the Whiteley Index has a three-factor structure (disease fear, disease conviction, and bodily preoccupation), more recent research suggests a unitary hypochondriasis dimension may underlie the scale (Speckens et al., 1996). Investigators have found the total Whiteley Index to have adequate test–retest reliability and internal consistency and to correlate highly with other measures of hypochondriasis.

THE UTILITY OF RESEARCH INSTRUMENTS IN CLINICAL PRACTICE

This chapter has reviewed standardized instruments for the assessment of somatization phenomena that are applicable in mainstream scientific research or clinical diagnosis. Such instruments are designed to meet the familiar psychometric criteria of validity and reliability. They yield either numerical values or an "in or out" decision for placement within a diagnostic category. Such instruments are congruent with the requirements of randomized, clinical trials that are the common currency of psychiatric research around the world.

We do not, however, assume an identity between the constructs of somatization and whatever the tests measure. Nor do we think that these instruments and the nomothetic assumptions that underlie them completely comprehend the various phenomena of somatization. All clinicians, even those applying manual-based treatments in the context of a research study, will inevitably recognize the uniqueness of each human being and the futility of attempting to capture the complexity of human beings with standardized research instruments.

Systematic idiographic, qualitative approaches to assessment abound in various quarters, from medical anthropology to phenomenological psychology. A discussion of these approaches that employ "alternative" methods, such as focus groups and ethnographic analysis, is beyond the scope of this book. Our emphasis on mainstream approaches does not bespeak an assumption of the epistemological superiority of the putatively objective methods with which the mainstream research culture is associated. Much of our clinical work is predicated upon the assumption that a psychotherapist knows his or her patient in manifold and nuanced ways, many of which elude the capacities of the standardized methods that gauge, evaluate, and depict individuals with somatization symptoms. Clinical observation is essential in the context of discovery and the formation of hypotheses. Virtually all our advances in psychotherapy have come from individual therapists thinking idiographically about what approach would benefit a particular patient. To test conjecture, a more generalizable methodology is required. Someday we may have scientifically cogent qualitative assessments of somatization that will operate in concert with the more mainstream quantitative measures.

CHAPTER 5

The Context of the Therapy

Chapters 5 through 9 describe the current and most comprehensive version of our psychotherapy for somatization. They present not only all aspects of the therapy included in the 10-session version, whose efficacy has been examined in two controlled clinical trials, but also some additional developments in the treatment. Affective cognitive-behavioral therapy (ACBT) for somatization is a work in progress. As this book has been written and rewritten, we continue to learn more about how to diagnose and treat our patients, how to train students in the therapy, how to collaborate with our patients' healthcare providers, and how to involve most effectively patients' families.

This chapter contains an introduction to the therapy we employ in our work with somatization patients. Here we set the stage, as it were, for the methods of treatment and describe such contextual factors as the framing of treatment, the therapist–patient relationship, and the interface of our psychosocial treatment with other kinds of healthcare received by the patient.

The first codification of the treatment was a 10-session standard-ized, "manualized" intervention, the manual for which is presented in Appendix A. The 10-session treatment is succinct and highly struc-tured. It comprises relaxation training, behavior modification, cogni-tive restructuring, increasing emotional awareness, and interpersonal skills training. It is an abbreviated version of a longer intervention that we now employ with somatizing patients. It originally was conceptu-alized within a broad-spectrum cognitive-behavioral model, with spe-cial emphasis on relaxation training and the modification of illness behavior and related cognitions. The treatment manual for the 10-session treatment presented in Appendix A is *not* intended to be a "stand-alone" or "turn-key" psychoeducational device that could be effectively employed by a healthcare worker who did not possess a background in the methods of psychotherapy employed, receive training in the application of methods, or have concurrent supervision. It was created to be the blueprint for a randomized, controlled clinical trial (described in Appendix B) that would allow the empirical evaluation of a brief, standardized psychosocial intervention for somatization disorder. The use of the resulting 10-session treatment is justified by the cost-effectiveness considerations that are ubiquitous in the contemporary healthcare landscape and also warranted by the results of empirical research (Allen et al., 2006; Escobar et al., 2006), but we nevertheless view the brief treatment as an abridged version of a more comprehensive form of treatment that may be required to produce clinically meaningful and durable results with somatization patients. Chapters 5 through 9 describe the methods used in the 10-session treatment package as well as those additional components employed in longer-term work with this population. These chapters comprise the current and most comprehensive version of our psychotherapy for somatization.

FRAMING THE TREATMENT

Although generalizations can be risky assertions, it is safe to say that patients presenting with multiple unexplained physical symptoms are not typical of psychologically minded psychotherapy outpatients, who present with explicit emotional problems. Many somatizers are quite resistant to the idea that a psychosocial intervention could be relevant to or helpful for their problems. Many are convinced that their problems have nothing to do with stress or psychological factors and that they are suffering from a disease that either has not been diagnosed or the nature of which is unknown to medical science. Their conjectures could be correct. An individual's willingness to meet once with a mental health practitioner is not tantamount to a commitment to undergo psychotherapy. Some patients state their doubts directly. Others reveal their reluctance to engage in treatment by failing to see an association between stress and their symptoms. A few approach the initial session receptive to a stress-management intervention, but their doubts surface later when they are asked to explore links between specific somatic symptoms experienced and concurrent thoughts and feelings.

The therapeutic posture we assume with patients and the rationale for treatment that we present to them are among the most important elements of our therapy. Our attitude toward patients is empathic and interested. We begin by asking patients about their physical symptoms and about the impact those symptoms have on their lives. Our questions about the particular nature of the symptoms, such as the types of pain (e.g., stabbing, pounding, burning, aching) and the situations in which symptoms typically occur, provide therapists with important information while concurrently validating patients' discomfort. Patients' beliefs about their physical symptoms and past coping techniques are also explored. Throughout this discussion and throughout the entire treatment, the therapist strives to acknowledge the physical symptoms and the distress associated with them. The therapist's efforts to validate the patient's discomfort and distress are critical to the development of therapeutic rapport. Because patients presenting with somatization symptoms are so accustomed to being discounted or dismissed by their healthcare providers, they often become more willing to engage in treatment after they feel understood by their therapist.

After communicating a considered appreciation of the patient's difficulties, the therapist describes the treatment's rationale. A biopsychosocial model of physical symptoms is proposed. Here, the therapist's stance is empathic and nonconfrontational. For patients who attribute their symptoms to an unknown biological mechanism or to toxic aspects of the physical environment, the therapist suggests that even if symptoms are caused by some organic pathology or by environmental agents, stress is likely to exacerbate them. In this way, the therapist aims to expand and to create variations in patients' explanations of their symptoms, but is careful not to contradict patients' beliefs directly. Faulty beliefs about symptoms are more effectively challenged in future sessions after some trust and credibility have been established.

When the issue arises as to what we think is wrong with our patients, we tell them we do not know. If their problems could be explained, they would not be talking to us; they have medically unexplained symptoms. Relying on this tautology is the safest and most prudent response. If we are asked whether we think their problems are psychological, we emphatically say no. We do allow that stress can affect the body and that the effects of stress are mediated through various nervous tissues, including those in the brain. We state that stress can exacerbate an existing illness or predispose one to develop an illness. Often, patients will push the discussion deeper:

PATIENT: I know I am sick. The doctors have given up on me, and now I am here. But I know this isn't in my mind. You don't get the kind of pain I have from being psychologically screwed up, and I don't think being psychoanalyzed is going to help me.

THERAPIST: I agree. We are not going to talk much about your childhood. We'll be teaching you some skills that may make your symptoms less severe.

PATIENT: But this is psychological therapy. Isn't the assumption that I have emotional problems and that's where my symptoms come from?

THERAPIST: Sometimes a treatment can be effective without our understanding why it works. This is the case with many medicines that have been shown to be effective for a variety of illnesses.

PATIENT: My doctors and my family think I am a head case, and me being treated by a shrink will prove it to them.

THERAPIST: I think of it more like stress management for patients with cancer, coronary heart disease, and hypertension, which is part of standard care now. The principal difference is that we know less about what causes your symptoms. But, as you are well aware, even when people have an established diagnosis, it is not clear that the diagnosed disease is the source of all their physical symptoms.

Although it could be argued that we sidestep or finesse the question of whether somatization syndromes have a psychological origin and that we may be disingenuous or sophistical in our framing of the treatment in the early sessions, we refuse to be drawn into any debate that is predicated on the mind–body problem. This is because we do not believe that dualism is either sound metaphysics or a therapeutically helpful way of construing the world. Furthermore, when there is a contest between an organic and a functional explanation for somatic symptoms, a patient committed to an organic explanation may possess an incentive for failing in a psychological therapy (i.e., the failure of psychotherapy can be taken as evidence that the symptoms are organic and not psychosomatic).

The treatment is described as stress management. The rationale presented is that because stress is likely to aggravate physical symptoms, the reduction of stress is likely to alleviate physical discomfort. Many patients are open to this idea and, indeed, some already believe that stress might have a physical impact on their bodily sensations or may have played a role in their underlying but unknown pathology. Most somatizing patients, however, would not accept the notion that their physical symptoms are entirely a "direct" product of stress. Therefore, it is important that therapists clarify that stress is only one factor contributing to patients' physical discomfort. The avowed aim of this treatment is, by limiting the adverse influence of stress, to give patients control over the aspects of their illness that can be controlled. Below is another response to a patient who is displeased with the treatment rationale:

> PATIENT: Are you trying to tell me my symptoms are all in my head? I promise you, I really don't want to feel this way. There are lots of things I've had to give up because of my pain. I don't play tennis or work in my garden because of it.
>
> THERAPIST: No, I don't think your symptoms are all in your head. I have no doubt that if you could simply snap your fingers and have your symptoms disappear, you would have done so ages ago. From what you've told me, I can see that your life has been diminished greatly because of your pain. The adverse consequences have been substantial. What I'm proposing is that there may be a portion of your pain that you can gain some control over. Now, I'm not suggesting that you can make it appear or disappear at will. But, let's take an example: a natural reaction to pain is to tighten the surrounding muscles, as if the body were trying to brace itself against the pain. Unfortunately, this added muscle tension is likely to increase the pain. So, if we can eliminate the portion of your pain that is aggravated by tension, your pain won't disappear, but it may be 25–50% better. Would your life be any different if you had 25% or 50% less pain than you have today?

By the end of the initial session, patients typically are willing to consider the rationale we present to them. Nevertheless, difficulties arising from the mind–body issue are likely to reappear in future sessions. As treatment progresses, patients may resist suggestions that changes in thought and behavior can influence their physical symptoms. Thus, it is important that the therapist listen for skepticism in future sessions and respond to it as suggested above.

During the course of therapy, especially if symptoms are alleviated, patients may become more attuned to the nuances and complexities of the biopsychosocial model of illness and its implications for their particular case. At such a point the terms of discussion may broaden somewhat:

> PATIENT: I really have been feeling a lot better since last week. Do you think expressing that anger toward my boss could have made that much difference in my GI symptoms?
>
> THERAPIST: Clearly when you started treatment, you were not what we would call "in touch with your feelings." We believe that increasing awareness of emotional processing, finding the most apt label for our feelings, and owning up to our emotions, is the way to go in enhancing overall functioning. Could your unexpressed emotions have been a factor in your gastrointestinal symptoms? Absolutely. Aspects of GI dysfunction can impinge upon nerves that cause pain. Also, nerve impulses from the GI feed back directly through the vagal nerve into emotional centers of the brain. The neural connections between the brain and the GI tract send signals in both directions, signals that we sometimes are not conscious of. It might be that your boss's treatment of you upsets your GI directly through that mechanism and that your anger is a "spin-off" of that physical process. We just don't understand the cause-and-effect relationships associated with every symptom. But we believe that self-awareness is a good thing and that emotional intelligence usually makes people healthier.
>
> PATIENT: But do you think my physical problems come from blocked feelings?
>
> THERAPIST: That might be one factor in a very complex process. The frustrating thing about this from a scientific and logical point of view is that you and I will likely never know for sure. But if you start feeling better and have gained a little self-knowledge and self-awareness to boot, then I will be satisfied.

Although somatization patients are reputed to be "difficult" and to be chronically dissatisfied with their healthcare, our own experience has been one of high satisfaction on both sides. We have now assessed and treated more than 200 patients diagnosed with disorders in the somatoform spectrum. Less than 10% of our patients have withdrawn from treatment prematurely, though many have begun with "attitude problems" and manifested the reputed resistance. On the whole, we have found these patients to be exceedingly grateful, cooperative, and even enthusiastic about the treatment they have received.

Why has this patient group, commonly regarded as truculent and disagreeable folk, been such a joy for us to work with? We have only anecdotal data, but our sense is that these people have fallen through the cracks in the healthcare system and consequently have not been well served by it. They come to us skeptical, demoralized, and expecting one more runaround. We offer them respect, validation of their suffering, and neither promises of cure nor demands for capitulation and resignation. Some of these patients report that they have been blamed for their symptoms and told that there is really nothing wrong with them. Others describe a chronicle of endless medical tests and expensive and painful medical procedures, all ultimately useless. We offer a third way, between capitulation and triumph. Our approach has some credibility and plausibility for those who have vacillated between excessive hope and total despair.

ESTABLISHING RELATIONSHIPS WITH PATIENTS' HEALTHCARE PROVIDERS

The collaborative relationship with other healthcare providers is established at the outset of therapy when the primary care physician or other referring physician is contacted to confirm the diagnosis and to coordinate care. The physician's diagnoses of the patient's physical complaints and the recommendations for treatment are reviewed. Ruling out organic factors is, of course, a crucial issue when patients present with unexplained medical symptoms. The last thing a psychotherapist wants to do is dissuade a patient from receiving proper medical treatment for a diagnosable and treatable disease.

Some 20 years ago Smith and his colleagues (1986b) developed an approach to intervening in somatization disorder that consisted entirely of sending a psychiatric consultation letter containing treatment recommendations to patients' primary physicians. The letter described somatization disorder and advised physicians to (1) schedule somatizers' appointments every 4–6 weeks instead of "as-needed," (2) conduct a physical examination in the organ system or body part relevant to the presenting complaint, (3) avoid diagnostic procedures and surgeries unless clearly indicated by underlying somatic pathology, and (4) avoid making disparaging statements, such as "your symptoms are all in your head." This intervention was somewhat effective in reducing healthcare utilization in these patients. The Smith intervention established the value of the principle of close coordination between psychosocial treatment and somatic medicine, and that principle is reflected in our approach to patients.

Physicians are busy people, and our experience is that they vary widely in the amount of time they wish to devote to coordinating our psychosocial treatment with their own medical interventions. Frequently a physician treating a patient with somatization disorder is pleased to have the help and share responsibility.

> STUDY THERAPIST: Hello, Dr. Castalano, this is Dr. Lesley Allen. Thanks for returning my call. I am treating your patient Susan Klein as part of a clinical trial funded by NIH. We are evaluating an intervention designed to reduce stress in medical patients. Did you receive her release and our letter of notification?
>
> PHYSICIAN: Yes, both are in her file.
>
> STUDY THERAPIST: First, I'd like to corroborate the diagnosis we have arrived at. A semistructured interview indicates that Susan qualifies for two DSM-IV diagnoses, somatization disorder and major depressive disorder. Would you agree with those diagnoses?
>
> PHYSICIAN: I have Susan on 100 mg of Zoloft q.d. [daily] for depression.
>
> STUDY THERAPIST: And the diagnosis of somatization disorder?
>
> PHYSICIAN: She seems to have quite a few psychosomatic symptoms.

Sometimes sharing information can be helpful to both parties.

> PHYSICIAN: Susan has been tried on several antidepressants, but does not tolerate them well.
>
> STUDY THERAPIST: Thanks. She didn't mention multiple trials of antidepressants to us. But she did indicate to me that she has stopped taking her Zoloft.

Rather early in the conversation with the patient's primary physician the therapist describes our psychosocial treatment approach with the aim of enlisting the physician's support of the treatment. The therapist also clarifies the meaning of the consultation letter.

> STUDY THERAPIST: Does the idea of a stress-management treatment for Susan's somatic symptoms make sense to you?

PHYSICIAN: She's been very stressed for as long as I have treated her. In fact I suggested yoga or meditation to her.

STUDY THERAPIST: Do you have any questions about what we are doing with Susan?

PHYSICIAN: I do have a question about the treatment recommendations. Are you suggesting that I increase the frequency of her appointments?

STUDY THERAPIST: It might work out that way, depending on how often you typically see her. The suggested structure is designed to minimize irregular appointments, especially to change a pattern of scheduling an appointment any time a symptom becomes troublesome. The underlying rationale is that regular visits may provide a structure in which she might be able to resist making unscheduled appointments.

THE THERAPIST–PATIENT RELATIONSHIP

Virtually all patients diagnosed with somatization syndromes have had extensive, unsatisfying, and futile encounters with the healthcare system. These patients always have failed to benefit from at least one previous intervention. The most common pattern is that our intervention is the latest in a long line of treatments, all of which have been failures. Given that their expectations are low, our patients must be motivated to come to therapy, despite minimal initial hope of success. Our patients tell us that what keeps them coming back is the opportunity to be treated by someone who cares about them and who makes a respectful effort to understand what their lives are like.

There is great debate in the psychotherapy literature about how crucial the therapy relationship is to the production of favorable results; some have even attempted to describe the proportion of outcome variance that is due to relationship factors (Norcross, 2002). In our work with somatizers it seems evident to us that the relationship is absolutely crucial. It is during the early sessions, before the benefits of the intervention are achieved, that the therapist–patient relationship is most important. Some patients have had previous experience in psychotherapy, but for many of them our treatment is their first time working with a psychotherapist.

In ACBT we place a great emphasis on psychotherapy as a caring encounter. We emphasize this to a greater degree than do many expositions of cognitive-behavioral therapy, a treatment that usually is associated with a didactic therapist–patient relationship, absent the emotional intensity of older, more traditional forms of psychotherapy, such as psychoanalysis or client-centered therapy. While it is true that in ACBT the therapist functions as a teacher and a trainer, he or she also is a confidant and a helper who must earn the patient's trust through being truthful, caring, and empathic. The kind of caring encounter that is based on genuine and sincerely felt compassion is essential to being effective with the patients we see. They have, in many cases, not been treated with kindness or courtesy. In the areas of civility and sympathy, our therapy often proves to be a corrective emotional experience. Caring and empathy are not, in themselves, sufficient to produce change in our patients, but they can be important elements in a restored sense of confidence in the healthcare system and in the resolution to attempt to cope with what can be great discomfort and disability.

CHAPTER 6

Behavioral Interventions

This chapter describes the behavioral methods we employ in our work with patients with somatization. We illustrate each behavioral treatment component, including relaxation training, increasing activities, pacing activities, reducing illness behavior, addressing sleep difficulties, and coordinating care with primary physicians.

RELAXATION TRAINING

More than 50 years ago, Joseph Wolpe (1958) produced an abbreviated form of Edmund Jacobson's (1938) method for reducing tension in the skeletal musculature. Since then, relaxation training has been a staple of behavior therapy. Other methods of lowering physiological arousal, such as paced respiration, biofeedback, meditation, and autogenic training, have been established by empirical research to be effective methods of managing some of the adverse effects of stress (Lehrer, Sime, & Woolfolk, in press; Lehrer & Woolfolk, 1993; Woolfolk & Lehrer, 1984). Some form of relaxation training is currently used in cognitive-behavioral therapy (CBT) for a number of stress-related disorders, such as panic disorder, generalized anxiety disorder, and tension-type headaches (Barlow & Craske, 1994; Borkovec & Costello, 1993; Holroyd, 2002).

In our work with patients with somatization, we use two forms of relaxation: diaphragmatic breathing (Fried, 1993) and progressive muscle relaxation (Bernstein & Carlson, 1993). Relaxation serves a number of functions in the treatment of somatization disorder. It may interrupt the muscle tension–pain cycle found in chronic pain patients (Linton, 1994). It may reduce generalized physiological arousal or physiological reactivity that has been observed in these patients (Rief, Shaw, & Fichter, 1998). Also, cognitive benefits may result from patients' observations that they are not completely helpless victims of their symptoms, but instead have some control over them (Lehrer et al., in press).

We employ relaxation training early in treatment because most patients report benefits from it soon after its initiation. Early gains in treatment may reduce patients' skepticism about the efficacy of therapy and facilitate their engagement in it. In order to ensure that patients master relaxation skills and incorporate them into their daily lives, the therapist devotes a significant portion of six or more consecutive sessions to relaxation training. We typically teach diaphragmatic breathing for the first month of treatment and an abbreviated progressive muscle relaxation (PMR) for the second month of treatment.

We begin with diaphragmatic (abdominal) breathing because it is easily learned, willingly practiced, and easily generalized to most everyday situations. Abdominal breathing can be implemented even in high-stress situations such as public speaking, childbirth, and competitive athletic contests. Breath control is a key element of many meditative and yogic traditions. Breath control methods in Indian hatha yoga include Dirgha Pranayama, which features what is equivalent to what we call diaphragmatic breathing. Also equivalent to diaphragmatic breathing are the breathing components of the "water method" of Qigong (Chi Kung), a set of traditional Chinese medicine practices that are analogous to yoga. Breathing deeply and slowly occurs, either advertently or inadvertently, in various forms of meditation (e.g., Zen meditation [zazen]) and in Western techniques of paced respiration or breathing retraining. Interventions that feature modification of breathing as the only active intervention have proved effective in ameliorating stress-related psychological and physical symptoms (Freedman & Woodward, 1992; Meuret, Wilhelm, Ritz, & Roth, 2003). Diaphramatic breathing can be used in concert with PMR. We subscribe to the view that relaxation training is most effective when it enables the trainee to learn how to relax on any given occasion and throughout the day, as opposed to extended sessions occurring once or twice per day during scheduled times when an especially deep state of lowered arousal is achieved.

The therapist introduces diaphragmatic breathing and explains that the long-term goal is for the patient to breathe abdominally as much as possible. Regular abdominal breathing, however, takes time to establish if it is a departure from the patient's typical practice. Over the course of treatment, the patient will be asked to practice breathing abdominally between sessions and to report back on his or her progress. Eventually, breathing abdominally may coincide with reductions in tension and discomfort, though the patient should be warned not to be disappointed if he or she initially experiences little significant relief.

To get started, the patient is instructed to set aside time to breathe diaphragmatically twice every day for 15 minutes. We typically warn the patient that a 15-minute interval may seem excessively long at first because (1) he or she may be unaccustomed to allocating time for such an activity, and (2) sitting quietly doing nothing but relaxing initially may seem like wasting time or a prescription for boredom.

It is important for the therapist and patient to work collaboratively in planning the time and place at which the patient will practice his or her breathing (e.g., in the kitchen before leaving for work). When practicing abdominal breathing, the patient should be in a quiet place where he or she will not be disturbed. Another strategy some people find helpful during the early phases of skill acquisition to facilitate training in diaphragmatic breathing is to practice while reclining, instead of while sitting. If the patient is having difficulties learning the abdominal breathing technique, the therapist may recommend practicing in a comfortable and familiar location, such as on the couch, in a reclining chair, or in bed. The guiding principle is that any correct practice, anywhere, is better than no practice.

After practicing diaphragmatic breathing at home for a few weeks, the patient is asked to breathe abdominally throughout one or more treatment sessions to develop increased awareness of the process of breathing and to begin learning to breathe abdominally while engaged in other activities. During these sessions the therapist interrupts the conversation every 5–10 minutes to question the patient about his or her breathing. If the patient is either unaware of his or her breathing or is aware that his or her breathing is not diaphragmatic, he or she is encouraged to stop talking for a few seconds and to refocus on diaphragmatic breathing. Although therapists may initially feel hesitant to interrupt the flow of the session to focus on breathing, we believe this practice has a powerful and salutary impact on patients. It teaches patients that they can begin to observe and alter their breathing patterns as they perform everyday activities. Our sense is that monitoring breathing during therapy can facilitate making abdominal breathing a part of patients' daily lives.

Additional strategies to help patients expand the use of diaphragmatic breathing in their lives are employed. First, the therapist encourages practicing diaphragmatic breathing in nonstressful situations, such as while watching television, reading, or bathing. Once the patient feels comfortable with and is calmed by abdominal breathing in peaceful situations, emphasis is placed on using diaphragmatic breathing during a wider range of daily activities. Mnemonic devices, such as placing "stickies" on computers, refrigerators, or mirrors and making calendar entries reminding patients to relax, may be recommended. Patients eventually are encouraged to use diaphragmatic breathing before and during stressful situations as well as in response to feelings of physical discomfort.

Our typical sequence of relaxation training is to teach diaphragmatic breathing until the patient has acquired some facility with its use and then to introduce our own abbreviated form of PMR. If after 2 weeks of training a patient has unusual difficulty with diaphragmatic breathing, finds it aversive, or does not enter a moderately relaxed state upon employing it, we shift to PMR immediately.

The method of PMR we employ is highly abbreviated from the Jacobsonian original method (Jacobson, 1938). Although our training is much briefer than Jacobsonian PMR, we do not employ some of the modifications that are commonly used by cognitive-behavioral therapists. We do not attempt to induce relaxation by having patients produce maximum muscle tension and then subsequently release that tension. This method proved to be impractical with patients with somatization because many of them suffer from pain in the skeletal musculature and have little tolerance for a strenuous tensing of muscles. Jacobson's original method uses minimal initial tension (and subsequently diminishing tensions) and focuses on teaching trainees to recognize and release small amounts of muscle tension. Our approach adopts this emphasis on awareness, discrimination, and letting go of tension, rather than on the production or suggestion of relaxation. The Jacobsonian expression "go negative" is used to describe the process of freeing the muscles from tension, of going limp or reducing muscle innervation. From the very beginning, we place an emphasis on patients' being aware of muscular tension throughout the day and using relaxation skills in those everyday situations where it is practical to do so.

We address 16 muscle groups, taken in groups of 12 (both lower arms, upper arms, lower legs, and upper legs are tensed concurrently). Patient training in PMR is described further in Appendix E. After doing PMR in session with the therapist's guidance, the patient is given a list of each targeted muscle group as well as systematic instructions on doing PMR at home (Appendix E).

Although some patients ask for an audiotape of the PMR instructions, we decline such requests with the following rationale based on Lehrer's (1982) analysis: When people practice relaxation by listening to instructions via audio media, they may never learn to self-administer relaxation. Becoming dependent on a voice recording, they may not learn to achieve acceptable levels of relaxation in the absence of externally administered instructions. Our aim, instead, is for patients to be able to use PMR at any time or place without requiring any aids or devices. Consistent with the overarching objective of treatment (to give patients as much control over their stress and physical discomfort as possible) we want to avoid fostering any dependence on external devices or other people.

The crucial challenge in relaxation training is helping patients use the techniques on a regular basis. The considerable amount of therapy time used to describe, practice, and implement effectively relaxation techniques indicates the importance we place on using them. Even though training in relaxation is often completed by the eighth week of treatment, we continue to inquire into patients' use of relaxation throughout our work with them. Some patients learn to use both abbreviated PMR and abdominal breathing, either in combination or separately. Others have a strong preference for one method or the other. We attempt to train patients in two forms of relaxation and to allow the patient to decide ultimately which to employ. At this point the research literature cannot demonstrate that any form of systematic relaxation is superior to others for a given individual (Lehrer & Woolfolk, 1993). What is clear, however, is that relaxation is beneficial only if it is utilized.

Based on this last assertion, it could be argued that optimally therapists should provide a wider set of relaxation alternatives with the expectation that if a varied menu of relaxation offerings is sampled, the patient is more likely to find one technique that will be to his or her liking and continue to be employed after treatment has ended. We have chosen diaphragmatic breathing and abbreviated PMR largely for reasons of clinical pragmatism. These are two techniques that are comprehended and learned readily, both by patients and therapists. In longer-term treatment, additional techniques, such as meditation or autogenic training, also may be taught.

BEHAVIORAL MANAGEMENT

Increasing Activities

Many somatization patients respond to their physical discomfort by withdrawing from activities that are potentially pleasurable and fulfilling, such as work, social activities, hobbies, and exercise. Illness behavior and the sick role may come to provide the organizing framework for these patients' lives. The behavioral module of treatment aims to increase gradually patients' vocational, recreational, and self-care activities and to improve their mood, self-esteem, and physical robustness. For example, unemployed patients are encouraged to engage in meaningful activities such as volunteering their time, taking a class, or doing favors for friends or family. Patients who have withdrawn from social activities are encouraged to reconnect with others by telephoning or e-mailing a friend, returning to church or temple, or joining a book club.

Behavioral methods are largely based on the principles of classical and operant conditioning. Existing pathogenic contingencies of reinforcement are replaced with salutary ones. For example, patients learn to connect with friends and family by engaging with them in pleasurable activities instead of interacting with them through activities focused on the patients' physical discomfort. Exercise assignments are designed to be pleasurable and commensurate with patients' physical capacities, so that exercise may eventually be reinforced by inherent natural contingencies. Overall, the acquisition of a broader repertory of activities also may serve to enhance each patient's self-efficacy in multiple areas and reduce feelings of infirmity and powerlessness.

The therapist begins this segment of treatment with a behavioral assessment. The patient is questioned about activities presently engaged in as well as about those avoided. The assessment also reviews activities carried out in the past. The therapist focuses on three categories of activities: meaningful activities (e.g., paid or volunteer work, household projects, education), pleasurable activities (e.g., social activities, hobbies), and exercise. (This is a loose practical taxonomy with the potential for categorical overlap.)

Next, the therapist provides a rationale for suggesting behavioral changes. The therapist says something like, "Many of our patients report they've stopped working, engaging in hobbies, or going out with friends because of their symptoms. And, although it makes sense to suspend activities that worsen your discomfort, if they aren't replaced with other enjoyable or meaningful activities you are left with a rather empty life." Once the patient accepts the rationale, the therapist works with him or her to consider the possibility of increasing pleasurable and/or meaningful activities. The importance of participating in some form of exercise that contributes to physical fitness also is emphasized.

To help a patient engage or reengage in an activity, the therapist examines and, if indicated, challenges the patient's thoughts about the activity. The advantages and disadvantages of engaging in the avoided activity, as well as the worst possible outcome of engaging in the avoided activity, are discussed. If the patient reports fears of an unpleasant outcome, the therapist should review the evidence supporting and contravening the patient's expectations. If the patient believes he or she would enjoy and/or benefit from engaging in the activity, the therapist asks what has interfered with the patient's participating in it.

Given that exercise improves mood, increases endurance and pain thresholds, and enhances sleep (Minor, 1991; Weyerer & Kupfer, 1994), we advocate exercise as one of the most important activities for patients to engage or reengage in. Many patients are not exercising when they begin treatment. (As described in Chapter 5, the therapist contacts the patient's primary care physician within the first few weeks of treatment. Recommendations to begin exercise are withheld until a physician provides medical clearance.) We first provide patients with a rationale for exercising: It reduces stress, improves the symptoms of chronic fatigue syndrome (CFS) and fibromyalgia, and improves mood. Also, the costs of not exercising include loss of muscle strength, the reduction of physical and psychological endurance, and the fostering and perpetuation of social isolation, negative feelings about self, and weight gain. Discussion focuses on the advantages and disadvantages of exercising for each particular patient. Below, a therapist encourages a patient to begin exercising:

THERAPIST: It sounds like you're busy professionally and socially. One set of activities you haven't mentioned is exercise.

PATIENT: Yeah. I had to give that up when my back and leg pain began.

THERAPIST: What kind of exercise did you do before?

PATIENT: I used to run with a running club. I was in great shape and loved being outside in the fresh air, even in the wintertime.

THERAPIST: Have you been exercising at all since you stopped running?

PATIENT: I tried walking, but it just didn't do it for me. So, I stopped. I am horrified with all the weight I've gained since then.

THERAPIST: If you were currently exercising, would there be any benefits?

PATIENT: Well, I'd probably lose some weight. But, I'm sure any exercise I would really enjoy would hurt my back.

THERAPIST: Okay. So, one advantage of exercising is weight control. You also indicated a couple of other advantages earlier: being outside and enjoyment. Two potential disadvantages are potential injury and lack of enjoyment. Let's make a note of these and also consider some other pros and cons of exercising. [The therapist and patient produce an extensive list of pros and cons, including those listed above.] So, it looks like there are lots of potential benefits from exercise if you could figure out a way not to injure yourself doing it. What do you think is the worst thing that could happen if you walked for at a moderate pace for 30 minutes three times per week?

PATIENT: It might be okay once. But, by the end of the week, I'd be bored to death and feel like I was wasting time.

THERAPIST: Is there anything you could do to reduce the boredom?

PATIENT: No. It's just dull.

THERAPIST: You mentioned that you used to run with a running club. Did you ever run alone, or were you always running with others in the club?

PATIENT: A couple times a week, I ran with the club. If not, I'd listen to my Walkman.

THERAPIST: Oh. Would it make walking more interesting if you walked with a friend or carried your Walkman?

PATIENT: I guess so. It's just such a pathetic form of exercise.

THERAPIST: Okay. So, perhaps the potential boredom is not the only obstacle here. It sounds like what's keeping you from walking is the belief that walking isn't real exercise. Is that right?

PATIENT: Compared with running, walking is nothing. I might as well watch TV.

THERAPIST: Well, let's take a closer look at that belief, that walking isn't real exercise.

Convincing patients to engage in avoided activities may require the use of cognitive restructuring techniques discussed in Chapter 7. As illustrated in the previous vignette, therapists help patients identify and challenge the beliefs that impede their activities. Once a patient expresses a willingness to engage in a new activity, experiments are designed to assess the effect of the change in behavior on the patient's mood and physical symptoms.

Activity Pacing

Activity pacing is an important topic to address when discussing the initiation of a new activity. Our clinical experience and some research suggest that some, if not many, patients with somatization have perfectionistic tendencies driving them to overachieve (Surawy, Hackmann, Hawton, & Sharpe, 1995; Ware, 1993). Our sense is that many of these patients may have difficulty moderating their activity levels; they overfunction at times and underfunction at other times. Of course, by the time they reach a psychotherapist's office, they are underfunctioning in important areas of their lives. Nevertheless, once they have been convinced to undertake an activity, they may be inclined to overdo it.

This overfunctioning/underfunctioning behavioral style is illustrated by one of our patients. Jane commenced treatment a few years after she had begun receiving disability payments in conjunction with a diagnosis of fibromyalgia. From her own and her husband's report, she rarely left her home except to attend appointments with physicians, of which she scheduled at least two per week. Yet, her physical appearance suggested a very high-functioning woman. Her hair was neatly styled; her makeup was carefully applied; she had flawlessly polished fingernails and toenails; and her outfits included matching jewelry, scarves, and handbags. When questioned about her daily activities, she acknowledged spending 2 hours "putting [herself] together" on days she left the house. She said that despite the fatigue and pain caused by her cosmetic activities, "I'm not the kind of person who can just throw something on and run out of the house. I like to have things just right."

Given the possibility that somatization patients may overfunction or strive for perfection in therapy, the therapist emphasizes the importance of making small changes in a specific behavior at first and subsequently instituting gradual increases in that activity over the course of therapy. If the patient fails to pace him- or herself, he or she is likely to overexert him- or herself, confirm his or her negative beliefs about the perils of being active, and become inactive again in the future. For example, if a patient has not exercised for 10 years, he or she should consider taking three short, slow walks (perhaps lasting only 5–10 minutes each) during the first week. Likewise, initial homework assignments for pleasurable and/or meaningful activities should represent small steps toward a longer-term goal. Although the therapist elicits the patient's suggestions for homework assignments, it is the therapist's responsibility to ensure that the weekly assignments are manageable. In deciding on an assignment, it is preferable to err by asking patients to do too little than by asking patients to do so much that they experience aversive overexertion or a sense of failure. If one week's homework assignment is insufficiently challenging, the assignment can be increased for the following week.

Another way in which activity pacing is incorporated into therapy is by persuading patients to take frequent breaks in the midst of their daily routines. Some patients are even encouraged to reduce the pace at which they carry out their lives. For example, one of our patients was an engineer who worked 50–55 hours per week for a small medical technology company. Claiming to be too tired and too distressed by burning sensations in his feet (a medically unexplained symptom) to engage in family activities or household projects, he spent much of his free time resting and watching television. When asked how he spent his time at work, the patient's feelings of pride and self-righteousness reflected his view that he was "keeping the company afloat," yet he barely disguised his fears of failure. In his words, "the intensity of my job is more than most people could handle." Though it was difficult to convince this patient of the potential benefits of slowing down at work, he eventually agreed to experiment with taking abdominal breathing breaks every hour and trying to work at 80% capacity (instead of his usual 100% capacity).

To increase the likelihood that behavioral changes become a permanent part of patients' lives, they are discussed throughout treatment. The therapist monitors all changed behaviors every week of treatment.

Illness Behavior

For expositional purposes, we will now discuss our approach to illness behavior, although we do not address this topic in treatment until the patient has learned some of the cognitive strategies described after this section.

One of the costliest aspects of somatizers' illness behavior is their excessive use of medical care. Patients who are overly concerned about their health may not be comforted when a medical examination fails to uncover a problem. In fact, they may selectively attend to and misinterpret physicians' reassurances. Alternatively, they may recall stories of acquaintances' medical conditions that were misdiagnosed for years before the discovery of a fatal disease. Hence, a physician's reassurances may prompt the seeking of second and third opinions. Repeated physician visits typically increase the patient's body-focused attention, hypervigilance, health anxiety, and emotional distress, all of which may increase his or her sensitivity to pain and amplification of symptoms. As this escalating cycle of increasing discomfort and physician visits continues, the doctor–patient relationship deteriorates in a predictable manner. Both parties tend to feel frustrated; the patient senses his complaints are not taken seriously, and the physician believes her time is being wasted with exaggerated, spurious physical complaints.

In hope of interrupting this dysfunctional pattern of physical symptoms that prompt physician visits that fail to resolve and possibly exacerbate those symptoms, the therapist helps the patient learn to reconsider the thoughts fueling illness behavior. Our patients often make comments like "there must be something wrong with me that my doctor hasn't found." If such a belief is sound, the rational response is to seek additional diagnostic procedures. Such beliefs may, however, be assailable. Patients are encouraged to look at the evidence that either supports or undermines that belief. Questions like "What makes you think there is something medically wrong with you?" or "What evidence is there that the doctor has missed something?" are followed by "What evidence is there that you *may not* have a serious medical problem?" Also, patients are questioned about the advantages and disadvantages of having another diagnostic procedure. They are asked what would convince them that they are *not* suffering from the illness they fear. The grounds for the falsification of beliefs are explored extensively to demonstrate that one can never be 100% certain of perfect health. In addition to challenging patients' beliefs associated with illness behavior, the therapist constructs behavioral experiments in which patients test the consequences of avoiding (or at least delaying) physician visits. Symptom-monitoring forms are used to assess the impact of modifying this aspect of illness behavior. If patients can delay a physician visit long enough, the somatization symptom that initially prompted the intent to seek medical treatment may subside.

In addition to including these direct interventions for illness behavior, the treatment may also indirectly reduce healthcare utilization by encouraging patients to increase meaningful and pleasurable activities. For some of our most severely impaired patients, the sick role and its associated help-seeking behaviors are the focus of their lives. Consider Sally, a patient who had retired from her job because of her fibromyalgia and irritable bowel syndrome (IBS). Her adult children no longer lived with her. Her husband worked full time and traveled frequently for his job. Refusing to eat at restaurants or at her friends' homes because of the intense gastrointestinal reactions she would experience after ingesting most foods, Sally also had withdrawn from her friends. Thus, she had no job, no caretaking responsibilities, nor any other daily meaningful or pleasurable activities. During the initial stage of treatment, Sally's only regular social contact was with her doctors. Each week she had at least two doctors' appointments in addition to her session with us. Her rheumatologist met with her once every week or two, her primary physician saw her monthly, and various other practitioners—including a gastroenterologist, dentist, chiropractor, gynecologist, and allergist—treated her regularly. A large fraction of her meaningful contact with other human beings occurred during appointments with medical practitioners.

Over the course of 3 months in treatment, Sally gradually began to experiment with expanding her range of activities beyond interactions with healthcare professionals. As a first step, we challenged her belief that she should not make commitments for social engagement because of the unpredictable and incapacitating nature of her physical symptoms:

> THERAPIST: Let's look at this concern you have, that you can't commit to an activity or event because your symptom flareups will force you to cancel frequently. In the past 2 months, how often have you cancelled your doctors' appointments?
>
> PATIENT: Well, I'm careful to schedule them in the afternoon, when I'm usually feeling better. So, I probably haven't canceled any recently.
>
> THERAPIST: As far as I can recall, you haven't canceled any appointments with me.
>
> PATIENT: Yeah. Doctors' appointments are important. Even if I'm having a tough day, I really try not to miss them.
>
> THERAPIST: Okay. That's interesting. If you schedule activities that you value in the afternoon, you're likely to follow through with them. Is there anything we've been talking about, for example, either volunteering or attending a book discussion group, that you could schedule in the afternoon and that would be important enough to push yourself to attend, even on bad days?
>
> PATIENT: I really would like to volunteer at the church. But I hate the idea of breaking my commitments. I also don't want to feel like I have to go if I'm in a lot of pain.
>
> THERAPIST: Well, maybe that's something we could experiment with. What would you think about making a small commitment to volunteer, say, 1–2 hours per week, and seeing how that goes?
>
> PATIENT: Could I bail out if I'm having a bad day?
>
> THERAPIST: The idea would be to make a small commitment and

treat it like a doctor's appointment. See what happens if you try to push yourself to keep this one commitment. We are not talking about a big change, only a couple of hours a week.

Over time, Sally began to increase her commitments to other people, eventually volunteering twice a week at her church's after-school program, taking walks with her neighbor, and attending a weekly book discussion group. Her increased level of activity left her with less time to schedule doctors' appointments. These activities and the associated social interactions began to replace her doctors' appointments as organizing structures for her life. Over the course of treatment, Sally's other illness behaviors, such as withdrawing from activities and relationships and retreating to her sofa or bed, were reduced.

Coordinating Care with Primary Care Physicians

The management of illness behavior ideally is done in concert with the patient's primary care physician. After speaking with the patient's physician, the therapist is better equipped to help the patient comply with his or her physician's medical recommendations. Patients are unlikely to follow medical recommendations that have been misunderstood, forgotten, or discounted. Given the brevity of many medical appointments, physicians often have difficulty obtaining full understanding or compliance with recommendations. Many physicians' recommendations are consistent with a systematic behavior modification approach. If the physician has recommended exercise or dietary changes, the therapist discusses and assists the patient in making these changes. If the physician has prescribed a medication regimen that the patient is not following, the causes for noncompliance are explored, and the patient is assisted either in following it or in communicating his or her medication issues with the physician.

During the later stages of therapy when illness behavior and the sick role begin to be discussed in earnest, it is optimal that the therapist and the primary care physician agree on the proper level of medical care for the patient. Thus, one goal of our therapy is to facilitate an effective working alliance between the patient and his or her primary care physician. There is always the possibility that a psychotherapist will be perceived as a meddler or that conflicting views of the patient's illness may emerge, but in our experience, such difficulties are rare. The key problems between somatizers and their physicians stem from poor communication and insufficient time allocated to the analysis of the patient's problems. Our experience is that physicians and patients usually are grateful to have another professional involved in monitoring, regulating, and augmenting treatment. Once the therapist and primary care physician have decided on an appropriate level of medical care for the patient's presenting symptoms, the therapist can challenge the patient's belief that additional medical treatment should be sought:

> PATIENT: I need to see a new doctor to find out why I don't have any energy.
>
> THERAPIST: Have things gotten worse in this area lately?
>
> PATIENT: I'm not sure. But I want to feel better and get some answers. Maybe a new doctor will have some new ideas.
>
> THERAPIST: Certainly this is possible. But for now it is vital to our work to stay with the original plan of scheduled visits to your current physician until we complete our work together. Part of what we are trying to do is break a cycle, a pattern of behavior. When you get frustrated, you go to see a new doctor. The anticipation of improvement temporarily raises your hopes, but the actual experience of consulting a new physician results in more frustration when you don't get any better. Meanwhile, you have intensified the focus on your illness and had one more unsuccessful experience with the healthcare system. If you have observed no decline in your energy level in the last week, I think we should stay with our plan.

We, as therapists, can feel confident in discouraging patients from scheduling new medical appointments only if we have established a collaborative working relationship with the treating physician and know the patient will meet regularly with the physician.

Addressing Sleep Difficulties

Many patients with somatization syndromes report significant sleep disturbance (Affleck, Urrows, Tennen, & Higgins, 1996; Morriss, Wearden, & Battersby, 1997; Roizenblatt, Moldofsky, Benedito-Silva, & Tufik, 2001). Failure to receive adequate restorative sleep is a contributory factor in exacerbating many psychiatric disorders. In somatizers, almost invariably, sleep loss is correlated with a worsening of symptoms. We now believe that treating insomnia early and aggressively is a key to successful treatment of somatization.

Many of our patients, especially those not working outside their homes, engage in problematic sleep practices that may increase the likelihood of insomnia, such as taking naps during the day, keeping erratic sleep schedules, and watching television in bed. To combat poor sleep habits, we provide patients with brief psychoeducational training in sleep hygiene and stimulus-control techniques. The therapist begins by conducting a detailed inquiry into the patient's sleeping habits. Training follows those suggestions recommended by Bootzin and Rider (1997) and Morin (1993). The basic guidelines for a streamlined sleep hygiene are the following:

- Get up at the same time every day, all 7 days of the week.
- Use your bed only for sleeping or sex. Don't watch TV, have stressful discussions, or spend time worrying in bed.
- Keep your bedroom dark and comfortably cool.
- Go to bed only when you are sleepy.
- If you're not asleep after about 20 minutes, go to another room and do something relaxing. Return to bed only when you are sleepy. Follow this rule for nocturnal awakenings.
- Don't drink coffee, tea, or alcohol within 6 hours of bedtime.
- Have a light snack before bed.
- Exercise regularly, but not within 4 hours of bedtime.

Facilitating adequate sleep may require coordinating care with the patient's physician(s). It may be necessary for sleep medication to be prescribed as a short-term intervention to remove the adverse effects of sleep deprivation and to assess the patient's functioning under conditions of adequate sleep. Although we are cognizant of the potential adverse consequences of dependence on soporifics, these costs must be weighed against the great benefits of providing the salutary impact of adequate sleep. We are currently involved in evaluating the impact of sleep medication as a principal intervention with somatization. Time will tell just how efficacious this component of treatment will prove to be, but pilot data appear to show considerable impact in some patients.

CHAPTER 7

Working with Cognitions and Emotions

In this chapter we offer a description of the cognitive therapy techniques we utilize and an elaboration of the experiential, emotion-focused components of treatment and the therapeutic assault on the patient's sick role. Training in emotional awareness and labeling of affect was a component of the original 10-session version of this treatment. We came to believe that, in order to be implemented effectively and used in conjunction with cognitive methods in a comprehensive program of emotional regulation, the emotion-focused methods should be expanded and made more central to the treatment. Also, in the 10-session version of the treatment, the various cognitive and behavioral techniques are implemented adequately, but the therapeutic attack on the sick role tends to be preliminary and rather limited, as is the case with our attempts in that format to make patients more emotionally self-aware. Our conclusion drawn from early work is that patients' comfort with emotional exploration, willingness to alter habitual patterns of illness behavior, and acknowledgment of secondary gains involved in the sick role are greatly facilitated by a trusting therapeutic relationship and hampered by a superficial, formal, task-oriented therapist–patient relationship. Both endeavors (i.e., exploring emotions and recognizing secondary gains) require substantial trust on the part of the patient, enough to make him- or herself vulnerable and transparent. The current, expanded treatment necessitates a more substantial and closer therapist–patient relationship than usually can be established in 10 sessions and, thus, assumes a longer period of contact between patient and therapist.

IDENTIFYING, EXPRESSING, AND MONITORING

The cognitive-emotional elicitation/regulation components of treatment aim to help patients differentiate and understand their thoughts and feelings so that they can interact more effectively with their environments. The atmosphere of sessions devoted to this enterprise is more psychotherapeutic and less psychoeducational than that of the earlier sessions focused on relaxation training and making behavioral changes. Cognitive and emotion-focused strategies (Greenberg, 2002; Kennedy-Moore & Watson, 1999) are integrated and individualized, using case-based formulations (Persons, 1989).

Patients begin this phase of treatment by monitoring their thoughts and emotions associated with changes in their physical symptoms. Experiential techniques, such as focusing (Gendlin, 1981) and techniques from Gestalt therapy (Perls, 1973; Stevens, 1971), are used to assist patients in attending to, identifying, labeling, accepting, and expressing their thoughts and emotions. In our experience, patients with somatization typically are disinclined to focus intensively on their emotional experiences, but they often are willing to explore emotions co-occurring with their physical symptoms and to try to make sense of those emotions by examining associated thoughts and behaviors.

Symptom-monitoring forms are introduced to help patients focus their attention on thoughts and feelings between sessions (see Figure 7.1). These forms are analogous to dysfunctional thought records used with depressed patients (Beck et al., 1979). Our symptom-monitoring forms require patients to describe two specific moments each day: (1) when their physical symptoms are relatively severe and (2) when their physical symptoms are relatively less severe and they are experiencing greater relative comfort. Because the goal here is to increase patients' awareness rather than to assess symptom severity, it is not critical that the patient write about "the most uncomfortable" or "the least uncomfortable" period of the day. We aim for a record of representative "physically uncomfortable" and "physically less uncomfortable" episodes. Ideally, these entries will be made as proximate to the time of occurrence as possible. On days without significant variation in physical discomfort, patients' instructions are to choose, retrospectively, episodes of relative comfort and discomfort. At the moment of recording, patients note the time of day, the physical symptoms experi-

	Date/Time	Physical Symptoms Rate the intensity (0–5).	Situation What were you doing at that moment?	Emotion What did you feel? Rate the intensity (0–100).	Thought What were you thinking about at that moment? What was going through your mind at that moment?
Uncomfortable moment					
Relatively comfortable moment					

Rating Scale for Physical Symptoms

0 = no physical discomfort
1 = slight physical discomfort, discomfort can be ignored
2 = mild physical discomfort, discomfort can't be ignored but doesn't interfere
3 = moderate physical discomfort, discomfort interferes with concentration
4 = severe physical discomfort, discomfort interferes with many activities
5 = very severe physical discomfort, discomfort requires bed-rest

Rating Scale for Emotions

0 = no experience of the specified emotion
1 = the slightest degree possible of the specified emotion
.
.
.
100 = the most intense experience of the specified emotion

FIGURE 7.1. Symptom-monitoring form (used in treatment).

enced, the environmental circumstances, and thoughts and emotions concurrent with the physical symptoms. The monitoring forms can be used to detect patterns in symptoms and in the relationships among symptoms, thoughts, and emotions.

Although patients complete symptom-monitoring forms in response to changes in symptomatology, the exercise is intended to increase patients' awareness of the situations, thoughts, and feelings that coincide with these symptomatic fluctuations. With this population's tendency to attend excessively to physical sensations, our aim is not to encourage additional "body scanning," but increased awareness of physical changes and of the psychosocial context in which they occur is helpful in ascertaining connections between symptoms and stress.

To demonstrate the use of the monitoring forms, the therapist guides the patient in completing one form for the previous day. First, the therapist asks at what time of the day the patient's symptoms were particularly aversive. A specific moment in time, as opposed to a block of time, should be selected for each occurrence of symptomatic distress. The therapist assists the patient in identifying and documenting the precise situation in which the symptoms occurred as well as the physical sensations, thoughts, and emotions experienced at that specific time. The intensity of each physical symptom experienced at that moment is rated on a 6-point (0–5) scale, and the intensity of each emotion experienced at that moment is rated on a 101-point scale (0–100). Afterward, the therapist and patient complete an entry for a moment during the previous day when the patient's symptoms were less intense.

Initially, patients must be taught to distinguish between physical sensations and emotions and to differentiate thoughts from emotions. For example, if a patient says that his or her physical sensations included anxiety, the therapist might reply, "I would consider anxiety an emotion, not a physical sensation. So, let's put that in the emotion column. But sometimes people have physical sensations that accompany anxiety. Did you feel anything in your body, any physical sensation, at that time that coincided with the anxiety?" Similarly, if a patient says that he or she felt stupid, the therapist should (1) label this experience as that of the evaluative cognition that "I am stupid," (2) distinguish between cognition and emotion, and (3) question the patient about the emotion that coincided with that cognition. Learning to differentiate among emotions is emphasized. (Patients are asked to use specific emotion terms such as "sad," "worried," or "annoyed," instead of more nebulous emotion terms such as "stressed," "upset," or "feel bad.")

Many patients presenting with somatization struggle with the self-awareness activities because of difficulties in identifying and differentiating among their thoughts and feelings. Whatever the cause of this difficulty (e.g., alexithymia, repressive coping), our efforts focus on enhancing awareness and acceptance of thoughts and feelings. Many patients find recognizing and expressing thoughts and/or feelings the most difficult component of treatment. Nevertheless, these initial skills must be mastered before cognitive restructuring techniques can be taught. Challenging cognitions is futile unless one can identify one's thoughts *and* feelings.

Some patients have trouble identifying thoughts and/or feelings in part because they have learned that they feel less distressed when they distract themselves from their thoughts and/or feelings. In fact, some patients become quite skilled at ignoring thoughts and/or feelings. If the therapist has evidence of an unacknowledged emotion (e.g., the patient expresses negative affect nonverbally by manifesting an angry voice tone and facial expression, but denies experiencing any negative affect), he or she should gently confront the patient in a manner like the following:

THERAPIST: So, what are you feeling about the argument with your mother-in-law?

PATIENT: I'm not feeling anything. But I will not be talked to that way. My mother-in-law is a not a nice person. She is a bitch, really.

THERAPIST: It sounds like you're having trouble identifying feelings. On the one hand, you said you don't feel much about the argument with your mother-in-law. On the other hand, while we've been talking about that argument, I've noticed your face turn red and your tone of voice sound irritated. I wonder whether you are aware of anything physical that you are experiencing right now, at this very moment.

PATIENT: No.

THERAPIST: You don't have to decide so quickly. Take a moment to tune into your experience of the workings of your body. Pay attention to your face and your neck and shoulders and your stomach.

PATIENT: Well, it does feel a bit hot in here. I may be sweating a bit.

THERAPIST: Okay. Did you feel that way when we were practicing abdominal breathing a few minutes ago?

PATIENT: Hmm. I don't think so. I just started noticing it since you asked me to focus.

THERAPIST: Okay. What do you make of the fact that you're feeling a bit hot and sweaty?

PATIENT: I guess I got a little worked up when talking about my wife's family.

THERAPIST: Worked up? Can you tell me how it feels to be worked up?

Initially, many patients will not be able to describe their feelings in any greater detail than the patient mentioned above. At this point, the therapist might give the patient the list of emotion terms (see Figure 7.2) and ask which of these terms best describes the way he is feeling.

Some patients have trouble identifying what they experience. These patients may respond with blank stares to questions like "What was going through your mind at that moment?" When this occurs, we attempt to elicit emotions in session with emotion-focused techniques, such as focusing, role playing, or using imagery to describe the situation in detail as if it were occurring in the present. Once the patient expresses his or her emotion(s), he or she is asked about his or her interpretations of the situation: "What does this [situation] mean to you?" or "What's bad about this [situation]?" Also, the patient's thoughts about the symptoms experienced in that situation might be explored: "What are you thinking about your [physical symptom experienced at that moment]?" or "What does it mean to you to have that [symptom] again?"

Sometimes the only thought a patient can associate with increased physical discomfort is a "coping" thought. Coping thoughts typically occur immediately following a more negative thought to which the patient may not have attended. For example, the patient experiences a headache, which he or she adds to the physical symptom column, and writes the thought, "I can handle this." In response to this recorded thought, the therapist might say:

THERAPIST: Let's go back to the moment you noticed your headache. You are hanging up the phone and you feel the stabbing pain in your temple. What goes through your mind next?

PATIENT: I can handle this.

THERAPIST: What do you say to yourself just before you think, "I can handle this"?

Afraid	Angry	Annoyed
Anxious	Ashamed	Bashful
Blue	Bored	Confident
Confused	Contemptuous	Content
Curious	Delighted	Depressed
Disappointed	Discouraged	Disgusted
Embarrassed	Enthusiastic	Envious
Excited	Frightened	Frustrated
Gloomy	Guilty	Happy
Hopeless	Humiliated	Inspired
Interested	Irritated	Jealous
Loving	Mad	Nervous
Proud	Relieved	Repulsed
Sad	Scared	Scornful
Shy	Surprised	Worried

FIGURE 7.2. List of emotion terms.

PATIENT: I don't know.

THERAPIST: Hmm. The thought "I can handle this" makes me think you're trying to reassure yourself that you won't be overwhelmed by the headache if it becomes intense.

PATIENT: Yeah. They can get really bad at times.

THERAPIST: Right. And that's pretty difficult when they do. So, it sounds like one of the ways that you've learned to cope with them is to reassure yourself. You're sort of your own coach or cheerleader, maybe. You remind yourself that you can handle them. Is that right?

PATIENT: I guess so. I hadn't really thought about it. There's not really anything to do.

THERAPIST: So, just before you think, "I can handle this," might you have a negative thought about the headache, such as "Oh no, not another headache"?

PATIENT: Probably something like that.

THERAPIST: Is it another thought, or is that the one?

PATIENT: No. That's it. It's like "not again."

THERAPIST: Okay, go back to the situation again. You're just hanging up the phone and you notice one of those bad, stabbing headaches. You think to yourself, "Oh no, not another headache." What does the prospect of a headache mean to you?

PATIENT: My day is ruined. I'll be miserable all day.

THERAPIST: So, those sound like the first thoughts that go through your head, even though the thoughts may not be fully articulated. And after having a quick sense or prediction of the day being ruined by the headache, you reassure yourself that you can handle it. Is that right?

PATIENT: Yes. That pretty well captures it, now that I think about it.

THERAPIST: Okay. This is what I'd like you to write in the thought column of the symptom-monitoring forms. I'm interested in the first thought, the distressing thought, the raw, uncensored one, the one you try not to focus on because it's upsetting. Or maybe it is difficult to capture because it goes by so fast or is replaced with the reassuring thought so quickly. [The therapist writes the thoughts "My day is ruined. I'll be miserable all day" in the thought column.]

PATIENT: I don't think I pay attention to my thoughts.

THERAPIST: I think you're right. You may have discovered that you feel discouraged or annoyed or even anxious when you focus on these sorts of negative thoughts. So you've learned to look for a positive response to these negative thoughts. My guess is that finding a positive response has helped you cope. I don't want to take that away from you. However, I may be able to help you find some additional coping responses if I know what the initial negative thought is. For a few weeks, I'm going to ask you to slow things down when a physical symptom occurs, to tune in to your inner workings, and to try to identify what you are thinking, even if the thought process turns out to be a negative one. Then write down the thought, with the expectation and understanding that you could feel a little worse initially while doing this. Again, the goal of this exercise is to provide you ultimately with more tools to cope with upsetting thoughts and feelings. Does that make sense to you?

It is useful to help patients identify thoughts that can be subjected to thought-challenging in future sessions. When emotions are embedded in thoughts, the therapist helps differentiate thoughts from feelings. The thought "I was pissed that he ignored me" is analyzed into a thought ("He ignored me and was rude in doing so") and an emotion ("pissed" or angry). The factual content (or value judgment) expressed by the thought "He was rude and unjustified in ignoring me" or its significance may be disputed. On the other hand, the emotion attached to that thought is not disputable. People feel whatever emotions they feel, whether those emotions are justified, appropriate, or are what they would like to be feeling.

For tactical therapeutic purposes, thoughts posed as questions are treated as rhetorical questions and transformed into assertions. If a patient records a question in the thought column such as "Will my back pain leave me bedridden?", the therapist should help the patient restate the question as a statement, such as "My back pain may eventually leave me bedridden."

To help detect the emotional intricacies of patients' inner worlds, the therapist should pay attention to whether moods and associated thoughts are congruent. For instance, sad moods typically correspond to thoughts about loss, anxious feelings usually correspond to thoughts about impending danger, and angry feelings generally correspond to thoughts about injustice or an infringement of rights (Lazarus, 1994). If the patient's thoughts are not congruent with his or her feelings, the therapist should ask for additional thoughts and feelings.

For example, a patient might write that his or her mood was "sad" and his or her thought was "It's not fair that I have this much pain and fatigue." The therapist should attempt to evoke thoughts that correspond with the "sad" feeling (e.g., thoughts about loss). Also, additional moods (e.g., anger) that correspond with the thought "It's not fair" should be investigated. In all such cases, the therapist should treat the patient as the ultimate authority and not attempt to impose a view on the patient about the presence or absence of a particular cognition or emotion in a reported situation. In the following example, the therapist attempts to find unstated thoughts and feelings:

THERAPIST: You are reporting the thought "It's not fair." When you have this thought, "It's not fair," I'm sensing there might be another associated emotion besides sadness. Consider that possibility for a moment. Let's focus on a thought here and now. Explore this thought to see if it matches your own thinking. Try it on for size to see if it fits. You're in more pain and are more fatigued than anyone you know, and you're only 35 years old. Can you think that thought here and now?

PATIENT: Yeah. I'm thinking it.

THERAPIST: How do you feel?

PATIENT: Sad, depressed.

THERAPIST: What else?

PATIENT: I don't know.

THERAPIST: Let's focus on the sadness for a moment. Usually, when people experience sadness, they are experiencing some kind of loss or disappointment. Have you experienced losses since your pain and fatigue started bothering you so much?

PATIENT: Everything. I had to quit my job because of how bad I feel. My social life stinks now because I'm too tired to do anything. I don't do anything!

THERAPIST: How do you feel now?

PATIENT: Sad.

THERAPIST: Okay. So those thoughts correspond with the feeling of sadness. Let's write that down. [The therapist writes, "I've had to give up my job and my social life because of this pain and fatigue."] Let's examine the thought "It's not fair." Experiment with saying to me "It's not fair."

PATIENT: You want me to say it to you?

THERAPIST: Yes.

PATIENT: It's not fair.

THERAPIST: Say it again, and say it a little louder.

PATIENT: It's not fair!

THERAPIST: Again.

PATIENT: It's not fair!

THERAPIST: Does that statement fit? Is that what you believe?

PATIENT: Yes. It isn't fair.

THERAPIST: Are you aware of your voice and your face?

PATIENT: Yeah. I'm pissed.

Although many patients may be unwilling to acknowledge feeling angry, they may own up to irritation, annoyance, or feeling "pissed."

Multiple treatment sessions will be spent reviewing monitoring forms to deepen patients' self-awareness. In these sessions, the therapist asks the patient to read aloud entries from his or her monitoring forms. The patient is encouraged to visualize, describe, and enact the events reported and to describe related thoughts, feelings, and symptoms as if they are occurring in the present moment. Here, the therapist emphasizes the patient's emotional experiences. The patient's attention is directed to his or her postural and nonverbal behavior as well as internal physical sensations during the session. For example, if a patient's arms are folded tightly around his or her waist, the therapist might say, "What are you doing with your arms right now?" The therapist might ask the patient to exaggerate that posture/activity by saying, "Can you hold yourself a little more tightly now? What do you experience now while you are doing this?" Also, the therapist observes and describes changes in the patient's voice, breathing, and facial expression and encourages the patient to verbalize associated feelings. When the patient expresses an emotion, he or she is asked to continue to focus on it: "Stay with that sad feeling for a few moments." This heightening of patients' self-awareness is facilitated by the therapist's refraining from challenging cognitions until a thorough investigation of emotions and their companion cognitions has been conducted. We want patients to be able to experience and communicate emotions during a session. This work in session is extended to the patient's life outside of therapy via homework assignments that call upon the patient to identify and record emotions and associated physical symptoms and thoughts.

Once a patient's unique pattern of cognitive and emotional responses is identified, a case-based formulation is used to guide treatment. Emotional elicitation may be emphasized to help assimilate previously disowned or disavowed cognitive and/or emotional experiences. For example, if it is agreed that the patient inhibits feelings of anger, portions of treatment sessions and homework may be devoted to facilitating the introspection, identification, labeling, and perhaps the expression of anger. Alternatively, emotional regulation strategies, including relaxation, distraction, and cognitive restructuring, may be implemented for dysfunctional, destructive, exaggerated, or uncontrollable emotions. Determining which emotions for a given individual in which circumstances need to be elicited or amplified and which need to be attenuated by examination through the lens of associated cognition is a task central to the integration of cognitive and emotion-focused methods. An example of a woman who experienced severe stomach pains after an incident at work follows:

PATIENT: I was treated very badly in a meeting at work on Wednesday. My boss implied that I was incompetent in front of our entire group. He did it in a particularly revolting, macho, sexist way.

THERAPIST: How did you feel?

PATIENT: I felt he was a jerk.

THERAPIST: "He is a jerk" would be an example of a cognition, an evaluative cognition expressing your opinion of him. What emotion were you feeling?

PATIENT: I was frustrated with the situation.

THERAPIST: Does frustrated mean irritated or annoyed?

PATIENT: Yeah, I guess so.

THERAPIST: I don't want to force you to guess. Please close your eyes for a moment and picture the scene you described where your boss denigrated you. Can you picture it?

PATIENT: Yes, I can picture it.

THERAPIST: What do you feel as you picture the scene? What is your emotional response to the scene?

PATIENT: I feel annoyed at my boss, but also bad about myself in front of all those people.

THERAPIST: That sounds like you may be feeling ashamed.

PATIENT: Yes, ashamed and humiliated.

In this example, the therapist asks the patient to bring a past event into the present moment, to experience it in the here and now through imagery and through the use of the present tense, as if the situation were occurring during the treatment session. Role-playing methods (Moreno, 1975) or the empty-chair method from Gestalt therapy (Perls, 1973) can be used to enhance emotional awareness.

Fritz Perls (1973) used to talk about the lack of affect clients feel when they "gossip" about past events, as opposed to bringing the events into the present moment by acting out and experiencing the event during a psychodramatization within the therapy session. For example, one patient appeared to be harboring feelings of resentment and anger toward her husband (Jeff), but could not seem to experience the feelings when talking about past incidents. The therapist asked her to do some role playing, to bring the situation into the "here and now" of the present moment, as opposed to relating stories from the remote "there and then" of the past. The empty-chair technique was utilized.

> THERAPIST: I'd like you to do a little role play. [The therapist places an empty chair in front of the patient.] I'd like you to imagine that Jeff is sitting there. Now he is obviously not really here to hear and remember what you say, so you can express your feelings without any consequences to your relationship. Can you try this?
>
> PATIENT: I don't know. This feels pretty weird.
>
> THERAPIST: Imagine that Jeff has just told you he wants to spend this Sunday watching football all day [a perennial issue between them].
>
> PATIENT: Yeah, he probably will. It seems selfish.
>
> THERAPIST: Remember he is here, in the chair. Look at him and tell him how you feel.
>
> PATIENT: Watching two football games when you don't even care about the teams involved in one of them is selfish. I don't like football.
>
> THERAPIST: What emotion are you feeling?
>
> PATIENT: That he is being selfish.
>
> THERAPIST: What emotion goes with that attitude?
>
> PATIENT: I'm just upset.
>
> THERAPIST: Tell him that then.
>
> PATIENT: I am very upset.
>
> THERAPIST: Let me give you a sentence to try on for size. Say to him, "I am annoyed with you."

PATIENT: I am annoyed with you.

THERAPIST: Again, this time a little louder.

PATIENT: (*Louder*) I am annoyed with you.

THERAPIST: Do those words fit your feelings?

PATIENT: Yeah, they do.

THERAPIST: Try this one: "I am angry."

PATIENT: I am angry.

THERAPIST: Does that fit?

PATIENT: Yes. I do feel anger.

THERAPIST: You feel it right now, toward Jeff?

PATIENT: Yeah.

Sometimes people have complex or seemingly inconsistent emotional responses. One can love and hate the same person. One emotion experienced can be accessible, while another, perhaps more primary, emotion is unavailable. Turning inward to introspect sensations as recommended by Gendlin (1981) can sometimes raise a complex emotional response to the surface.

Angela was a college professor at a major research university. She had earned tenure narrowly 3 years earlier. Angela had been troubled by numbness in her extremities, tinnitus, and severe menstrual pains. She was also subject to panic attacks. She complained about her job and her colleagues, constantly indicating that they did not take teaching or the welfare of their undergraduate students seriously; these were to her grievous faults. Angela was usually disappointed in her relationships. Sometimes the therapist surmised that Angela was critical of the therapy and of the therapist.

THERAPIST: So, then, are you feeling angry at your colleagues?

PATIENT: More miffed than angry, but a low level of anger, maybe.

THERAPIST: Let's try to explore this. When is your feeling of being miffed the most intense?

PATIENT: Probably at faculty meetings. That's when the prima donnas really strut their stuff.

THERAPIST: Okay, close your eyes, please, and try to picture yourself at a faculty meeting. Imagine someone is strutting his or her stuff.

PATIENT: All right. I am seeing it.

THERAPIST: Don't forget to breathe. It is very important that you breathe while you imagine this scene. Really let yourself be there. What do you feel?

PATIENT: Same old stuff. Waste of my time. These people think they are God's gift. A bunch of narcissicists.

THERAPIST: Tune in to what you are feeling. Focus on your body. What sensations are you feeling?

PATIENT: Some tightness in my chest and shoulders.

THERAPIST: Survey your entire body, head to toe. What are the sensations?

PATIENT: My throat feels uncomfortable. I feel like I need to swallow, but I can't.

THERAPIST: Is there an emotional tone to this set of sensations?

PATIENT: I don't know.

THERAPIST: You don't look angry now.

PATIENT: I feel bad.

THERAPIST: What kind of bad feeling do you experience in this moment?

PATIENT: I don't know. Sad, maybe. But like I want to run away.

THERAPIST: Afraid?

PATIENT: No, more like ashamed.

Angela had regarded her struggles to gain tenure at her university as fearsome at times, but principally she was aware of anger at her colleagues and her university. It proved to be the case that she also felt humiliated and shamed by the lengthy process of evaluation that assistant professors undergo. She did not like her colleagues but also had some reservations about herself.

DISTRACTION

As discussed in prior chapters, patients with somatization have a tendency to focus excessive attention on their bodies and to amplify their physical sensations. Our clinical observations have revealed that many patients experience their worst discomfort when they withdraw from activities and focus their attention on their physical symptoms. The goal of distraction is to help patients shift their focus away from their physical sensations.

We encourage the therapist to approach the discussion about distraction with discretion. Some patients will take offense to the implication that their physical symptoms are not so overwhelmingly intense that distraction would be possible. Others will say that they already spend much of their time distracting themselves from their never-ending feelings of discomfort. The therapist should persevere nevertheless and emphasize that one's focus of attention may influence symptom intensity. Furthermore, if one's symptoms are severe enough to prompt one to rest and focus on the symptoms, negative thoughts and feelings about the symptoms are likely to arise. These thoughts and feelings about the symptoms may, in turn, exacerbate them.

Some patients may distract themselves excessively at times and focus their attention too much on their physical sensations at other times. One of the patients we described earlier in Chapter 3, Rahim, the computer programmer, illustrates this pattern. While at work he was unaware of his thoughts, feelings, and physical sensations, whereas at home he directed inordinate attention to his physical sensations. We encourage therapists to help patients identify both the aforementioned patterns of (1) excessive attention to physical symptoms and (2) inattention and insensitivity to bodily sensations. (Note that we discourage patients from complete inattention to bodily sensations, a stance that could pose risks of overexertion and injury.)

Prior to the session in which distraction is discussed, the therapist reviews the patient's symptom-monitoring forms to determine whether the patient has reported feeling physically worse when focusing on his or her symptoms. If there is evidence of overfocusing on physical symptoms, the therapist brings this evidence to the patient's attention after acknowledging the patient's efforts to push through the pain at other times.

If, during the session, the patient acknowledges the pattern of symptoms worsening when he or she is especially "body-focused," the therapist and patient create a list of distracting activities. Examples of distracting activities include phoning or e-mailing a friend, reading an engaging novel, playing with a pet, doing mental arithmetic, writing a grocery list, and planning a trip. After completing the list, the therapist should ask the patient if he or she would be willing to attempt any of these activities over the next week instead of lying on the couch or in bed and focusing on discomfort. The therapist encourages the patient to think of this assignment as an experiment, a method to be attempted and evaluated. The patient can endeavor to use one or more of these activities on a trial basis between sessions and report his or her response during the following session. A typical discussion about distraction is transcribed below:

PATIENT: When my stomach starts acting up, it ruins my whole day. I just keep thinking about it, trying to figure out how bad the bloating and pain will be.

THERAPIST: What if we tried an experiment, approaching it another way?

PATIENT: What do you mean?

THERAPIST: Instead of focusing on the bloating sensations and pain, assessing their severity, and having your thoughts center on their adverse effects, what if you simply engaged in another activity, preferably something pleasant?

PATIENT: It's hard to enjoy anything when I get really bloated.

THERAPIST: I understand what you're saying. But, once the bloating and pain begin, the question is: Are there actions that may make it more or less tolerable? What would you think about getting on the Internet and planning your upcoming winter vacation the next time the bloating hits you?

COGNITIVE RESTRUCTURING

As summarized earlier, patients with somatization syndromes tend to have dysfunctional beliefs about somatic sensations and often about their ability to perform effectively. Also, most patients exhibit dysfunctional thinking about non-health-related topics. Sometimes, patients' cognitive errors cause them to act in ways that exacerbate their pain and discomfort. For example, one woman's rigid belief that "good friends should do whatever they can to help each other" prompted her to run herself ragged in the evenings and on weekends as she aided her friends.

An important component of treatment is to help patients examine their cognitive tendencies. After reviewing a few weeks of a patient's symptom-monitoring forms, the therapist will have a sense of the patient's typical dysfunctional thinking patterns. Cognitive errors that we have observed include perfectionistic thoughts, catastrophic thoughts (about physical symptoms as well as other life events), overestimating the possibility of negative outcomes, "should" statements, and dichotomous thinking. Our sense is that at the core of these errors is a global negative perception of self as being inadequate or unlovable. Although many patients may not acknowledge seeing themselves as inadequate or unlovable, especially within the 10-week horizon of the manualized brief treatment, thoughts about being weak, vulnerable, undesirable, unattractive, or helpless may not be far from the surface when the meaning of a thought is explored.

One note about labeling the cognitive-restructuring exercise for patients: We have found that some patients react negatively when their thoughts are described as "irrational" or when we suggest "disputing" their thoughts. Patients may interpret these labels as demeaning. To avoid such reactions, when speaking to patients about cognitive restructuring, we describe this activity as examining thoughts "more deeply" or "from different perspectives."

To begin teaching cognitive-restructuring skills, the therapist selects one of the patient's beliefs illustrating one of his or her cognitive tendencies. Next, the therapist and patient examine the thought from different perspectives. First, the patient is encouraged to find evidence supporting his or her belief. Then, evidence contrary to the belief is pursued. Behavioral experiments may be conducted to collect such information. One thought that we have challenged with many patients is the idea that any form of exercise will exacerbate their symptoms. After considering the evidence supporting and refuting this belief, we plan an experiment in which the patient engages in a few brief episodes of moderate exercise, such as taking a few 10- to 15-minute walks.

Another approach to helping patients look more objectively at their thoughts is to ask them to consider what they would tell a friend (or family member) who had similar beliefs in a similar situation. A mother who worked full time and did all the cleaning and cooking for her family stated, "a good wife and mother is responsible for all the housework. If I ask for help, I have failed." When asked to consider the advice she would give her daughter if her daughter tried to combine work and family, she was more willing to reconsider her rigid, demanding standard.

Another set of questions for the patient involves a pragmatic, cost–benefit analysis of having the belief: "What is the effect of believing that thought? What happens when you have that thought? What would happen if you didn't think that way?" As described earlier, thoughts about having a serious disease are likely to create significant feelings of anxiety. Examining the effects of such thoughts, including introspection of associated emotions, physical sensations, and behaviors, can be eye-opening to patients.

For "awfulizing" or catastrophic thoughts, the therapist encourages the patient to "assume the worst," to consider what is the worst that could happen if the belief were true? Could the patient live through it? These questions often expose the awfulized situation as inconvenient or undesirable, but not disastrous. When the catastrophic thought evokes a symptom's potential lethality ("This headache is a sign of an as yet undiagnosed but lethal brain tumor"), however, this line of questioning tends to be anxiety-provoking and unproductive. A more salutary set of questions is framed in terms of the evidence for and against the belief.

Together, the patient and therapist discuss and record responses to questions interrogating the rationality and impact of the patient's dysfunctional beliefs. Below is one example of such a discussion:

PATIENT: I had a very bad episode on Saturday. My fibro [fibromyalgia] was acting up.

THERAPIST: What was happening? What were the circumstances?

PATIENT: I was preparing for a visit from my children and grandchildren. It stresses me out. There is so much to do.

THERAPIST: Sounds like a lot of pressure. What if you didn't work as hard, what would happen?

PATIENT: Preparing a big dinner is a lot of work. They all have their favorite dishes. I want it to be special like it always was.

THERAPIST: What's the effect on you, to think the dinner has to be really special?

PATIENT: Ahhh. I get so tense and stressed.

THERAPIST: What if you cut the project down to size? What if you could be less perfect?

PATIENT: I don't think they would be happy. They wouldn't understand.

THERAPIST: What about you? Could you be satisfied with a less elaborate, superlative family event?

PATIENT: It would be hard to scale back.

THERAPIST: Would you feel less tense and stressed out if you didn't have to serve the perfect meal?

PATIENT: Maybe.

THERAPIST: Maybe some of the stress is coming from your own internal standards.

Some patients have trouble identifying a thought to challenge. A good rule of thumb is to select a thought that is associated with an intensely felt negative emotion such as feeling furious at a friend in a certain situation. The patient should consider the thought that evoked the anger. Questions like "What was so infuriating about that situation?" may reveal a disputable thought. Good targets for challenge and disputation are thoughts associated with a negative emotion that the patient believes to have been excessive or an overreaction. Thus, if the patient believed he or she felt disproportionately worried about something, the thought activating the worry would be a likely target for restructuring.

For homework the patient is asked to examine more deeply (i.e., restructure) thoughts that have recurred on the symptom-monitoring forms. The patient and therapist can identify recurring thoughts collaboratively during a therapy session. In addition to challenging specific thoughts, the patient will be asked to continue using symptom-monitoring forms to track physical symptoms and associated thoughts and feelings. If the patient finds any of the ensuing week's thoughts to be particularly distressing, he or she can examine them more deeply with the list of questions on the Examining Thoughts handout (see Appendix F).

The therapist should warn the patient that, like abdominal breathing, examining thoughts and attempting to modify them in this way is a skill that takes time to master. The therapist should inform the patient that this technique has been found to be extremely helpful for patients with chronic fatigue syndrome, irritable bowel syndrome, and chronic pain. Thus, even though it will feel awkward or inconvenient and perhaps even seem like a waste of time, the patient should be told that there is much research indicating that this approach to cognition can be very helpful. In time, the patient may not need to record his or her thoughts and rational responses to them. The process will become automatic. During the initial phase of learning to look more objectively at his or her thoughts, however, the patient should record his or her responses to each question.

CHAPTER 8

Interpersonal Methods

This chapter discusses what we have chosen to group into the category of "interpersonal methods." The interventions discussed here involve modifying the sick role, increasing assertiveness, and conjoint sessions with significant others that seek to intervene in and modify patients' home environments.

DISCUSSING THE SICK ROLE

The goal of discussing the sick role is to provide patients with some insight into any secondary gain they might derive while experiencing pain or discomfort and to examine the possibility that illness behavior has become habitual. Having identified the secondary gain, the therapist and patient collaborate to find alternative methods for attaining the sick role's benefits. For example, if the patient's spouse is especially nurturing when the patient is in pain, we help the patient ask directly for more attention and affection.

Examining the sick role's benefits is a sensitive issue because family, friends, and physicians may have accused the patient of faking, imagining, or exaggerating his or her symptoms. Thus, the therapist is careful not to imply that the patient is choosing to experience symptoms. The discussion will be fruitless if the patient becomes defensive. Because of the sensitivity of this topic, we typically defer its discussion until the eighth session of treatment.

To avoid raising the patient's defenses initially, the discussion begins by focusing on the patient's perceptions of other people who have been ill, people whom the patient knows or has known well. The therapist asks who, in the patient's family and social circle, had health problems during the patient's childhood (or during the patient's adulthood, if no one had health problems during the patient's childhood). In our clinical experience, as in the research of Craig, Cox, and Klein (2002), many patients meeting criteria for a somatoform disorder report having observed illness during childhood in either a family member or a close friend. The patient is asked to describe the individual who was ill and to talk about the ways in which that person's life was affected by illness or physical discomfort. Specifically, the therapist asks about the sick person's missed opportunities and missed experiences and how others responded to the person. Next, the therapist inquires into the "silver lining" that being unhealthy may have had for the sick person: "Were there any benefits of being unhealthy for that individual?" If the patient believes there were no benefits, the therapist may ask specifically about each of the following possible benefits: receiving special attention or nurture, avoiding undesirable activities, avoiding arguments, gaining a special role in the family, or diminishing one's own expectations for oneself. Usually, the patient will acknowledge that the ill individual experienced some benefits from his or her illness.

Having discussed another person's experiences with illness, the therapist shifts the discussion to the impact of illness on the patient's life. The therapist begins with inquiries into the patient's experience of illness as a *child*: "How did others respond to you when you were sick or in pain as a child?"; "Were you taken to the doctor or did you miss school when you were sick?"; "Did you receive special attention or treatment when you were sick?" Afterward, questions focus on the impact of illness during the patient's *adult* life: "In previous sessions we discussed the many disadvantages of your health problems these days. Are there any advantages to being sick?"

Although almost all of our patients have acknowledged that some benefits accrue from being sick, therapists often feel anxious during this discussion, especially when patients respond defensively. It may seem likely that explicit discussion with the patient about the sick role will undermine the therapeutic relationship, but in our experience, no patient has withdrawn prematurely from treatment after discussing the sick role. Although the topic is a sensitive one, it can be productively examined. The most common obstacles we have encountered during discussions of the sick role and our recommendations for the therapist are described below:

1. The patient denies knowing anyone who had a chronic health problem during the patient's childhood. In these cases, patients are questioned about their parents' and siblings' health: "Did anyone have chronic minor health problems, such as asthma or migraines?" Some patients will deny that any family members experienced even minor health problems. A patient who experienced no illness in his or her family while growing up may have been reared in a family that valued toughness and stoicism. Such patients may have come to believe that succumbing to illness is a sign of weakness.

If the patient has not known anyone with chronic health problems, the therapist moves from the discussion about others' health problems to the patient's own experience of illness. If a "never give into illness" message was communicated, the therapist should ask the patient how he or she feels about him- or herself, given his or her family of origin's values regarding health and illness. Also, the patient's current thoughts and feelings about others who are ill are explored: "How do you react to other people when they are ailing?"

2. The patient denies that there are any benefits that result from her health problems. When this occurs, the therapist should tread lightly while proceeding with the rest of the discussion; the patient may have begun feeling threatened by the subject matter. The therapist does not intend to suggest that the patient wants to experience discomfort or that the advantages of physical discomfort outweigh the disadvantages. Yet, in our experience, despite the many costs of physical symptoms, there are usually correlated benefits. As an illustration, the therapist may remind the patient of the benefits experienced by the ill individual from the patient's past discussed earlier in the session (if the patient identified someone else with health problems). Even if the patient could not identify any benefits of the sick role that accrued to the person from the past, the patient may have observed benefits that derived from his or her own childhood illness, such as kind treatment, special attention, gifts, missing school, or avoiding chores. Also, the therapist may suggest that some adult patients experience benefits during illness, such as attention or nurture, avoiding undesirable activities or arguments, gaining special status, or allowing one to "ease up" on oneself. If the patient continues to deny that there are any benefits of his or her health problems, the therapist shifts from a discussion of the sick role per se to a consideration of the broad topic of assertiveness.

Often the discussion of the sick role begins to provide a rationale for assertiveness training as it may reveal deficits in the patient's assertiveness. If the patient is deriving substantial attention or nurture through being sick, he or she also may be deficient in the ability to ask directly for attention and nurture. Patients who avoid undesirable activities by being sick may have difficulty setting limits on others. One advantage of the sick role is that people can be rewarded without having to ask directly for what they want. The sick role tends to undermine assertiveness and to provide few opportunities to hone skills of self-assertion, except perhaps in interactions with healthcare providers.

If the patient acknowledges that the sick role has become "second nature," we may borrow a technique of fixed-role therapy (Kelly, 1955) and have him or her attempt to play the part of a healthy person in one or more activities. One method is to ask the patient to find a role model who is not impaired and to imitate that person's behavior. Another is to have him or her ask the question "What would a healthy person do in this situation?" and then act out the answer. Occasionally, as much psychological research has shown, changes in attitudes and emotions will follow changes in behavior rather than preceding them. Expanding the range of the patient's behavior before the patient feels "healthy enough" can be effective if the approach is used judiciously. How much to push patients with somatization to extend themselves is a matter of clinical judgment. Good therapeutic decisions in this area tend to optimize treatment outcomes.

TEACHING ASSERTIVENESS

At this point in treatment, the therapist will have assessed for deficits in the patient's assertiveness. Some patients effectively assert themselves and have their needs met in some, but not all, situations. Some patients can assert themselves only in regard to certain kinds of needs. Other patients can assert their needs when they are aware of them, but may not always be aware of what those needs might be. Other patients have pervasive, traitlike deficits in assertiveness in virtually all areas of their lives. In our experience, all patients with somatization have difficulty expressing their thoughts and feelings assertively in at least some situations.

The therapist begins by defining assertiveness and explaining the rationale for helping the patient act more assertively in some situations. We define assertiveness as an open and honest expression of one's thoughts and feelings that avoids blaming or attacking others. Much of affective cognitive-behavioral therapy (ACBT) treatment, up to this point, has provided the groundwork for becoming assertive. For example, the self-awareness exercises and symptom-monitoring forms direct the patient to pay attention to his or her thoughts and feelings.

Stage 1 of acting assertively involves identifying thoughts and feelings. Stage 2, valuing one's thoughts and feelings, is implicit in and fostered by some of the behavioral techniques. By taking time to relax and to engage in pleasurable activities, patients are, in effect, affirming the value and legitimacy of taking care of themselves.

Before introducing Stage 3 of assertiveness, patients may need additional work on Stages 1 and 2. Specifically, patients might be asked to track their thoughts and feelings when interacting with others between therapy sessions. (At this point in treatment, unassertive individuals often can identify their thoughts and feelings when they are alone, yet they may have difficulty being self-aware while interacting with others, especially others who are accustomed to or expect them to be unassertive.) A homework assignment might be to ask, "What do I think and feel?" during various interactions with others. For patients who continue to have trouble valuing their thoughts and feelings, the therapist should use the technique from fixed-role therapy (Kelly, 1955) described in the previous section of this chapter. Patients are directed to role-play in the outside world, to behave as they would if they really did think their feelings and needs were important. Through this device, assertive behavior with a tone of conviction can be practiced and its often successful results can be witnessed by the patient. Occasionally, patients will adopt and assimilate features of this more assertive persona.

Stage 3 of assertiveness involves communicating one's thoughts, feelings, desires, and needs with "I" statements. The therapist suggests the patient use the following statement as a model, "I feel ___(emotion)___ when you ___(behavior)___." An example of content in this form is "I felt worried when you didn't call to tell me you'd be late coming home from work last night." By making such a statement, this individual is taking responsibility for his or her feelings as opposed to blaming others (e.g., "You're so selfish not to have called"). The statement is also indisputable since it is an expression of the patient's emotional reaction. The result is that the person being spoken to is somewhat less likely to react defensively than if attacked or explicitly criticized and may be less likely to attempt to refute the assertion itself.

"I" statements involving feelings are not natural or comfortable for many people to make. We typically do much role playing in session to help patients practice speaking assertively. First, we identify a recent situation from the patient's life in which he or she could have made an assertive statement. Details of the discussion are elicited. Next, we role-play the situation with the therapist playing the role of the patient and making assertive statements to the patient, who plays the role of an interlocutor. Afterward, we reverse roles, with the patient playing

him- or herself and speaking more assertively than he or she did originally. The therapist may give the patient suggestions for improvement
and ask the patient to replay the situation (sometimes repeatedly).

After role-playing some assertive statements in session, the therapist and patient identify a hierarchy of situations, from easiest to most
difficult, in which the patient could make assertive statements. For
example, saying no to one's spouse may be very difficult, whereas saying no to a salesperson may be relatively easy. Homework assignments
that require the patient to begin acting assertively are created and
assigned. The therapist also provides the venerable caveat that increased assertiveness on the patient's part may not be welcomed by
everyone. Increasing assertiveness effectively requires a consideration
of the impact of assertive behavior on other people and a judicious
weighing of the costs and benefits.

INCLUDING THE SIGNIFICANT OTHER
IN TREATMENT

The goals of including the significant other (domestic partner or
spouse) in treatment are to obtain additional information about the
patient, to gain the significant other's support for the treatment, and to
alter behaviors of the significant other that may reinforce the patient's
symptoms or illness behavior. We view this aspect of the treatment to
be so valuable that, even when working within our 10-session treatment format, we ask the patient's significant other to join us for one to
three of those 10 sessions.

We typically invite the significant other to participate in a conjoint
session within the first month of treatment. The rationale for meeting
together with the patient and significant other is to encourage an open
dialogue. In our experience, the therapeutic relationship is not always
strong enough to tolerate a therapist's meeting separately with a significant other, as some patients readily become suspicious that others
are minimizing their degree of discomfort. Although we would like to
begin deriving the benefits of including the significant other in treatment as soon as possible, for logistical reasons we typically delay the
first conjoint session until we have had some time to develop rapport
with the patient. We find the third or fourth session works well as an
initial conjoint session.

The conjoint session(s) includes discussions about the rationale for
a stress-management treatment and about how such a treatment could
be maximally helpful to the patient. The therapist asks the significant
other to comment on the impact of stress on the patient's physical

symptoms Also, the impact of the patient's physical symptoms on the patient's and significant other's lives is examined. Here we aim to elicit information and to suggest that the significant other's involvement in treatment may benefit both parties. Reducing the likelihood that the significant other will undermine the treatment is critical. Our aim is to prevent discussions like the following:

> PATIENT: Honey, can you try to avoid coming into the bedroom for the next 20 minutes? I'm going to go do my abdominal breathing.
>
> HUSBAND: You've got to be kidding. That stuff won't help you. Don't waste your time. Come watch TV with me.

After clarifying the treatment's rationale, the therapist attempts to determine whether the relationship with the significant other has been impaired by the patient's illness. The tendencies of patient with somatization to withdraw from activities may not only diminish pleasure in their own lives, but also in their significant others' lives. When a patient foregoes couple activities, such as eating at restaurants, going to movie theaters, dancing, or hiking, both the domestic partner and the relationship may suffer. The patient and significant other are asked to think about activities they once enjoyed and might yet again enjoy together. Afterward, the couple and therapist collaborate to develop a plan for increasing pleasurable conjoint activities. Reengaging in these activities may increase satisfaction with the relationship as well as reduce the patient's focus on his or her symptoms.

> THERAPIST: Thanks for coming in. I wanted you to join us for several reasons. First, I wanted you to have a sense of what the nature of the therapy is and to address any questions or concerns that you might have. Second, since you have lived with Jessica [the patient] during the entire time that she has been symptomatic, I thought it might be helpful to get a sense of your perceptions of and reactions to her difficulties, as you have witnessed them and been affected by them. Third, I wanted to make sure that we are all on the same page. The work that Jessica and I are doing together will be much more successful if you are on board and supportive of the treatment. Are there things you want to tell me or questions you have?
>
> HUSBAND: I have a lot of questions. I want to know if Jessica is going to be able to do normal things again. I want to know if we are ever going be like we were again.

THERAPIST: So this has been hard on you too?

HUSBAND: Well, you take what comes. But it's no walk in the park. It's been worse for her.

THERAPIST: But no walk in the park for you?

HUSBAND: That's right.

A subsidiary aim of the conjoint sessions is to address the couple's *communication* about the patient's physical symptoms. Initially, the therapist asks the couple to describe a few recent discussions about the patient's physical symptoms. Both members of the couple are asked to describe what each said about the symptoms and what each thought and felt at that time. Afterward, the therapist summarizes and reflects on the couple's communication about the patient's symptoms and provides suggestions for alternative modes of interacting that are less likely to reinforce illness behavior.

Some of the dysfunctional communication patterns that we have observed between patients with somatization and their significant others are described below. Our recommendations for addressing these communication patterns in a brief treatment are also provided.

1. Some significant others seem emotionally distant except when the patient complains of pain or discomfort, at which times the significant other is attentive, nurturing, and supportive. When the significant other's attentive behavior rewards and appears to reinforce the patient's illness behavior in this way, two recommendations are made. First, the therapist asks if the couple is willing to avoid the topic of the patient's health in their conversation. As an alternative to talking about illness, the couple is encouraged to discuss other topics of interest as well as to engage in pleasurable conjoint activities. During session, the couple and the therapist generate lists of possible discussion topics and pleasant leisure-time activities. Both members of the couple must be interested in the discussion topics and activities or willing to give each a try, so that they will both feel engaged in the activities. In theory, these alternative discussions and activities provide opportunities for companionship that is not illness-based.

2. Some patients seem to complain about their health during or immediately before unpleasant activities or conversations. Because of these complaints, a significant other may allow the patient to avoid the activity or discussion. This interpersonal dynamic demonstrates another way in which spousal behavior may reinforce the patient's illness behavior (e.g., complaining about health). When situations arise in which the patient is inclined to complain about a symptom in con-

nection with avoiding an aversive event, he or she is asked to refrain. Instead, the patient is asked either to endure the situation or to find an alternative reason for avoiding the situation.

3. Another interpersonal dynamic involves a significant other who ignores the patient when the patient complains about discomfort, leaving the patient feeling hurt and/or angry about his or her significant other's withdrawal. This interaction pattern may prompt the patient to escalate his or her illness behavior by complaining more, increasing time spent resting, and/or seeking attention from friends and medical practitioners. For this interaction pattern, the significant other is encouraged to acknowledge the patient's discomfort without overdramatizing it. In addition, the couple schedules some time each day to discuss non-health-related topics during which the significant other is expected to be attentive and supportive.

> THERAPIST: If we can, let's try to examine what happens in the relationship when Jessica's symptoms become severe. Either of you can tell me what happens, in general, or give me a specific example.
>
> PATIENT: Ed [the husband] is helpful, most of the time. He is very understanding. Sometimes he gets a little angry but most of the time he is supportive.
>
> THERAPIST: Ed, what do you do when Jessica's pain is bad?
>
> HUSBAND: I'll get her some tea or a diet soda. When she has to go to bed I'll take over with the kids. Sometimes I'll rub her feet.
>
> THERAPIST: Are you ever less supportive when she is in pain?
>
> HUSBAND: Well, she's right. Sometimes I do get pissed. Like when I had tickets to a concert last year and we couldn't go. She told me to go without her, but I couldn't leave her like that. We stayed home, but I lost it. Got annoyed. You know.
>
> THERAPIST: Did you communicate your annoyance to her?
>
> PATIENT: He yelled at me.

[The relationship between Jessica and Ed was what one might call a low-intensity, almost emotionally indifferent relationship. The most intense intimacy, positive and negative, seemed to occur in relation to Jessica's symptoms. Because the treatment was to be brief, the therapist chose not to confront the couple with this observation, but rather to begin to devise alternative opportunities for intimacy that did not revolve around Jessica's symptoms.]

TERMINATION AND REVIEWING SKILLS

In the case of the 10-session treatment, because the length of treatment is brief and its duration has been discussed repeatedly with the patient throughout the treatment, termination usually is less traumatic than in long-term, open-ended treatments. Nevertheless, many patients experience some sadness, worry, and even frustration at termination. The therapist should elicit and supportively reflect on the patient's thoughts and feelings about termination. If the patient reports irrational thoughts about termination (such as "I'll fall apart without you"), the therapist can guide the patient through a challenge of that cognition. The patient should be reminded that any improvement experienced during treatment is primarily a function of the patient's efforts between sessions. Also, the therapist can reassure the patient that many patients completing this brief treatment experience even greater improvements in the months and years immediately after treatment (if they continue to use the techniques learned). Thus, the expectation is for continued improvement, not relapse.

Whether patients are treated with our brief 10-session therapy or with a more extended intervention, the treatment aims to help them make changes in their lifestyles that will persist once treatment ends. Throughout treatment, as each skill is mastered, patients are pushed to incorporate the skills into their daily routines. As treatment concludes, the therapist places an even stronger emphasis on maintenance. In the last session(s), patients are questioned about situations in which they used each technique and about the impact of each technique on their symptoms. A plan for using each technique in the future is elaborated. Also, the patient is taught to recognize the warning signals that his or her thoughts or behaviors are regressing to former states and that former patterns of illness behavior are returning. Examples of warning signs are: (1) the patient has called in sick to work more than once in a month, (2) the patient's tic in his or her eye returns, (3) the patient spends a weekend day on the couch. Having identified potential warning signs, the patient and therapist plan strategies for altering the patient's behavior in response to such potential developments.

The possibility of additional treatment is discussed. Additional therapy may come in the form of follow-up or booster sessions. Other patients express an interest in pursuing additional treatment for other issues that were not addressed either adequately or at all in this treatment. The therapist can discuss referrals for additional treatment, if indicated.

CHAPTER 9

Assorted Clinical Topics

In this chapter, we describe various issues that are not essential to an exposition of the treatment, but that constitute the context or background of treatment. We also discuss assorted variations on the core themes of therapy.

PATIENTS, NOT CLIENTS

We refer to the people we treat as "patients" rather than "clients." This is not our own preference, which might incline in the opposite direction. The decision comes from polling the people we are treating and responding to their clear preferences. For most of them, the "patient" label connotes more nurture and caring than the more impersonal descriptor "client" and its associations with the worlds of law and business. Our charges are accustomed to being treated in medical settings in which the label "patient" is applied to all people with somatic problems. In fact, many prefer to conceive our treatment as a medical, stress-management intervention rather than an intervention addressing psychological issues.

THERAPIST TRAINING

The ideal clinician to implement our treatment would be an intelligent, empathic individual with training both in cognitive-behavioral therapy (CBT) and experiential psychotherapy, at least 5 years' experience in conducting psychotherapy, and exposure to most forms of adult psychopathology. Of the 20 or so individuals whom we have trained thus far to implement the treatment, none has met all the above criteria. For the most part, however, our trainees have proved to be very effective in working with patients with somatization. What, then, are the most important prerequisites?

In implementing the 10-session protocol, therapists need to be rather task-oriented and disciplined. Discussions with patients cannot be too open-ended; there is not enough time to "go with the flow" of therapy. Therapists trained in other forms of manual-based CBT or in brief psychodynamic therapy come to our work with a sense of the form, structure, and pace of the therapeutic endeavor. Therapists who have no experience in time-limited therapy may find somatizers difficult patients with which to be initiated into the practice of brief therapy. Patients with somatization often present with multidimensional and refractory problems and severe comorbid psychopathology, along with a vaunted truculence and obdurateness.

Perhaps the most difficult tasks in the treatment are the cognitive and emotional awareness exercises. Virtually all of our patients have trouble identifying and distinguishing between thoughts and feelings, cognitions and emotions, but we also find that those of our trainees whose only therapeutic training is in CBT do not always have great facility in parsing cognition and affect. This is why we suggest that some training in both experiential therapy and CBT would be a plus. We find trainees with a background solely in CBT may be insufficiently attuned to emotional nuance and less than optimally dexterous with labeling and exploring affects and allowing clients to experience their emotions. When establishing connections between cognitions and emotions, we want therapists to linger long enough with the affect to understand all the different feelings that may be associated with a pattern of thought. For example, if there is anger, that anger may be secondary to feelings of hurt, sadness, fear, or shame. Contemporary training in CBT can produce either a kind of tendentious stance toward the patient's dysfunctional cognitions or a proclivity toward premature validation of the patient's feelings, validation that is attempted before adequate understanding is achieved and sufficient empathy is demonstrated. In our treatment, we are cultivating emotional intelligence in our patients. We are attempting to help them understand and value their feelings as important indicators of who they are and how they react to the world. Some negative affects are highly dysfunctional and have little or no benefit, but others are crucial to patients' self-knowledge and need to be explored, experienced, understood, accepted, and sometimes communicated. A policy of rushing to cognitions in order to change them is inimical to our approach.

MEDICAL KNOWLEDGE

Implementing our treatment does not require medical training, but knowledge of the body and of those organic diseases with symptoms that are similar to the complaints of somatizers is very valuable. Inevitably, work with somatizers provides a kind of informal medical education. The patients themselves often provide highly elaborated medical-sounding explanations for their symptoms that may or may not be accurate. The diagnoses most frequently reported by our patients (though often subsequently disconfirmed by treating physicians) have been migraine headaches, osteoarthritis, and gastroesophageal reflux disease (GERD). Some background knowledge in psychophysiology, especially in stress and its physiological effects, is very helpful both for understanding patient complaints and in providing explanations to patients.

MEDICATION

Although research on pharmacotherapy for somatization thus far has yielded little in the way of highly successful treatments, studies currently being conducted may provide stronger evidence for the benefits of pharmacological intervention. In clinical practice, antidepressants often are prescribed under the assumption that they may ameliorate pain as well as help with mood and sleep. Among the antidepressants, empirical evidence for pain reduction is strongest for amitriptyline. There is growing interest in and data supporting the use of serotonin/ norepinephrine reuptake inhibitors (SNRIs), such as duloxetine and venlafaxine, for somatization syndromes (Arnold et al., 2004, 2005; Gendreau et al., 2005; Kroenke et al., 2006). The newer anticonvulsants, such as gabapentin and pregabalin, have recently become a popular treatment for fibromyalgia because of their safety and reputed sedating qualities. There is a small but growing body of evidence supporting the efficacy of these agents for neuropathic pain conditions (Pappagallo, 2003) and for fibromyalgia (Crofford et al., 2005).

Many somatization patients are treated with various pharmacological agents. Antidepressants are often prescribed for concurrent depression or anxiety as well as for pain. Anxiety and insomnia may be treated with tranquilizers and hypnotics, most commonly benzodiazepines, zolpidem, and eszopiclone. Pain may be treated with over-the-counter or prescription medications (e.g., narcotics, nonsteroidal anti-inflammatories, anticonvulsants). Also common is the use of gastrointestinal agents (e.g., laxatives, antidiarrhetics, antispasmodics, H_2-blockers). Therapists will want to be familiar with their patients' medications as well as the indications for these medications.

We recommend that therapists talk to patients as well as patients' physicians about the medication regimen. For those patients who are treated by multiple physicians who prescribe different medications, the clinician may want to help coordinate care. Therapists can assess patients' compliance with their medication regimens and patients' perceptions of their medications' effects. Some patients may be taking medications that have negative, as well as positive, effects. For example, pain relievers may exacerbate patients' gastrointestinal symptoms while alleviating various pain symptoms. The use of acetaminophen may reduce headache pain in the short run, while making additional headaches more likely. Opiates and tranquilizers may be misused and abused. Not only do we suggest inquiring into the somatic effects of medications, but we also ask patients about their thoughts and feelings about their medication use. Negative beliefs may influence medication compliance and, thus, may be targets for change in therapy, as well as a topic to be discussed with the prescribing physician.

RESISTANCE AND NONADHERENCE

As we discussed in the earlier chapters, patients with somatization often exhibit some resistance to the treatment rationale and some nonadherence to treatment. Therapists we have trained respond to resistance and nonadherence by communicating empathy for the patient's distress and discomfort while urging the patient to consider alternative perspectives and to experiment with new behaviors. As stated earlier, we have found many somatization patients to be less resistant than reputed, especially after trust and credibility are established. The feedback we have received from patients suggests that the affirmation, respect, and concern we evince toward them evoke, in many, an appreciation that translates into their putting forth effort to make changes. Some patients are so frustrated with standard medical treatment that an alternative approach is welcome. Some, however, dismiss the possibility that making behavioral or cognitive changes could reduce their discomfort. Skepticism of this kind can foster resistance and/or nonadherence.

Because resistance can be an elusive notion, we restrict our analyses and discussions to the less theory-laden notion of noncompliance. Noncompliance typically rears its head in discussions of homework assignments. Noncompliance with in-session activities is more likely to arise during the emotion-focused component of treatment and its potentially embarrassing role-playing and Gestalt therapy techniques.

As has been discussed throughout the behavior therapy literature, an essential element of using homework effectively in therapy is the therapist's follow-up on it. It is critical to discuss patients' experience with every homework assignment in the session that immediately follows the one in which the out-of-session project was assigned. When therapists fail to review assignments, they imply that the homework was not important and that future homework assignments also may be disregarded. As a general rule, when patients fail to complete a homework assignment, we spend a portion of the following session collaboratively completing some portion of that assignment or discussing the obstacles interfering with its completion (with the intention of minimizing them in the future).

A second widely held assumption about homework in therapy is that homework assignments that are designed collaboratively between patient and therapist are more likely to be completed than those designed by the therapist alone. Making changes in one's behavior is difficult. Compliance with suggested changes may be increased by encouraging patient input into those changes. For example, when a patient is asked to begin using relaxation or to start exercising, he or she should participate in deciding where, when, for what duration, and how frequently the activity should occur.

Homework compliance also may be enhanced by asking the patient to imagine and anticipate carrying out the activity. The therapist should ask questions: "What will it be like tomorrow evening when you sit down to breathe diaphragmatically? Where will you be? Where will everyone else in your family be? What thoughts will be running through your head?" Before leaving the therapist's office, the patient should discuss potential impediments to the completion of the assignment; when potential obstacles are identified, the therapist and the patient plan how to avoid or overcome them.

Even when homework is designed collaboratively and discussed in detail, some patients will not complete it. After ensuring the patient understands the rationale for the assignment, the therapist can ask the patient to consider the pros and cons of completing the assignment. Sometimes the therapist can persuade a reluctant patient to try a bit harder to do homework. The following tactics are sometimes helpful:

1. *Use the short-term duration of treatment* (e.g., "It's now or never"). In time-limited versions of the treatment, patients are reminded that treatment will end after the specified period of time, after which they are unlikely to benefit from these strategies if they have not implemented them during the course of treatment.
2. *Remind patients of their history of medical treatment:* "Nothing else has worked."
3. *Remind patients of the time and effort they already are expending on therapy.* Making a partial commitment to therapy may not be sufficient to derive the expected benefits from it. In fact, in some instances we have suggested patients might be better off not coming to therapy appointments at all and instead using that time to breathe diaphragmatically or exercise.
4. *Encourage patients to think of homework as experiments.* Patients are sometimes willing to agree to modify their behavior for a limited time, 1 or 2 weeks, as opposed to making a lifetime commitment. At the end of the specified time frame, they can reconsider the basis of their reluctance and noncompliance.

THERAPIST FRUSTRATION

There are a sizable number of pejorative labels that healthcare professionals use to refer to patients with somatization, such as chronic complainers, problem patients, and malignant personalities. These labels reveal the feelings of frustration and helplessness experienced by clinicians who work extremely hard to relieve symptoms that are resistant to change. If patients' symptoms fail to improve, patients themselves become frustrated and complain to their treating professionals. Some patients may even blame their healthcare workers for their lack of improvement.

Our approach has been to attempt to see the symptoms, not the patients, as the challenge. We must admit that this strategy is not always successful. It helps to have reasonable expectations and to work toward improvement but to expect no cures.

A clinician accustomed to working with more traditional patients in psychotherapy might experience all patients with somatization as defensive and resistant to introspection and perhaps start blaming them. If this happens, the best strategy for the therapist is to challenge his or her own dysfunctional cognitions and to resolve to empathize with the patient's discomfort— "to feel *his* or *her* pain." Therapists usually should assume the patient is doing the best he or she can.

DISABILITY

Many patients with severe and chronic somatization symptoms have difficulty fulfilling their employment obligations. Some pursue disability. We take the stance that long-term disability is not beneficial for our patients. Indeed, we regard it to be antithetical to our aim of restoring patients to the fullest possible range of life activities. The absence of a meaningful and productive life trajectory can be a contributory maintaining factor in somatization. Disability payments represent a financial incentive for maintaining the sick role. People adapt to disability, as they do to inactivity or to lack of structure or accountability. Restoration of functioning after a long period of subsidized disability is a very difficult clinical challenge.

When patients ask us to write a letter of support for their disability cases, we refuse as a matter of policy. We state that, instead, we would like to help patients increase their activity levels. Our aim is to support patients without supporting the sick role. Some patients will begin therapy after they have already been granted long-term disability. In these cases, we aim to help patients become more active in meaningful activities. Ideally, the goal would be a change in their disabled status.

HISTORY OF TRAUMA
AND PSYCHIATRIC COMORBIDITY

As discussed in Chapter 2, some patients presenting with multiple medically unexplained symptoms also report a history of trauma. Some of these patients are willing to address their past. For those who report feeling distressed about their history of abuse, we recommend CBT that includes exposure to the trauma, an approach not covered in this book. For those who decline to tackle their traumatic past, we conduct our treatment as outlined herein.

As discussed in previous chapters, the majority of somatization patients meet DSM-IV criteria for additional psychiatric disorders, typically depression and/or anxiety disorders. Such clinical complexity presents the psychotherapist with a decision as to whether to target somatization or the other psychiatric disorder(s). We recommend commencing treatment with a comprehensive psychosocial evaluation, including a medical history review. At the conclusion of the assessment, we ask patients what symptoms are most distressing to them and interfere most with their lives. Patients' responses to these questions determine the focus of treatment.

GROUP TREATMENT

As reviewed in Chapter 2, CBT for somatization syndromes has been conducted in group as well as in individual formats. In the only study comparing the efficacy of group versus individual CBT for these patients (a study of patients with irritable bowel syndrome), neither modality outperformed the other, while each appeared to be more efficacious than the control treatment (Vollmer & Blanchard, 1998). Apparently, individual and group formats both have therapeutic power.

In recent years, we have begun to combine our individual treatment with a group intervention. Our conceptualization and development of group treatment has been based on two kinds of considerations, each of which we view to be important: therapeutic efficacy and cost efficiency. Although ultimately, from a public health cost–benefit perspective, it would be important to determine whether group treatment for somatization might benefit patients as a stand-alone intervention, we have placed our emphasis on the utilization of group treatment in concert with individual treatment for maximum therapeutic impact. We think it is appropriate for patients who have received an initial course of our individual therapy to participate subsequently in group therapy. This practice is not unusual; referral to group therapy after individual treatment has been a common clinical practice for many decades. In the case of our particular patient population, the group format may lend itself especially well to reinforcing and maintaining therapeutic gains made by patients who have received individual treatment for several reasons.

First, patients with multiple medically unexplained physical symptoms have impaired social relationships (Zoccolillo & Cloninger, 1986). These patients may feel misunderstood by physicians and family members who often minimize the patients' discomfort and impairment. Psychotherapy groups consisting exclusively of patients diagnosed with somatization syndromes potentially can provide a supportive interpersonal context wherein patients can express feelings, compare experiences, and receive feedback from people with similar problems. Patients with somatization tend to feel isolated and unique in their maladies. They describe feelings of alienation because "no one understands" their physical complaints. Forming relationships with other people who do not regard the somatizer's experience as unusual or abnormal can be validating to patients.

Second, social reinforcement has a powerful influence on behavior. In group therapy, when patients report making adaptive changes in their behavior, group members are likely to be encouraging and supportive. Positive reactions from peers may promote subsequent adaptive change. Also, group norms that foster making therapeutic changes tend to develop. Peer pressure to change and even proscription of noncompliance serve as therapeutic incentives and disincentives.

Third, group members may serve as models of functional behavior for each other. Research suggests that models who are similar in characteristics such as age, sex, and appearance are more likely to elicit behavior change than models who are dissimilar (Bandura, 1986). Group members may, as role models, facilitate salutary actions more effectively than do therapists, who may seem less similar to patients than do other patients.

Fourth, a therapy group may serve as a microcosm of the client's interpersonal world. Group members may praise, offend, slight, criticize, or nurture each other. Examining and exploring such interactions, especially with regard to the cognitions and emotions elicited, can be therapeutically valuable. For clients who have difficulty expressing their emotions in the outside world, the group can provide a relatively safe environment in which initial efforts at more open and authentic expression can be made. Through receiving feedback and support from group members, patients also develop greater effectiveness in their interactions with family, friends, coworkers, and healthcare providers.

Fifth, an essential component of affective cognitive-behavioral therapy (ACBT) is teaching patients to examine their thoughts and reasoning processes for evidence of irrational assumptions or modes of inference (Beck, 1976; Ellis, 1962). In group ACBT, patients are able to examine their cognitions based on input from other group members. Group members can help each other identify and challenge dysfunctional beliefs. Here, patients serve as additional sets of eyes and ears as they function in adjunctive therapeutic roles. Often, feedback from group members is viewed as more impartial and objective than that provided by the therapist.

Finally, group theory maintains that interpersonal difficulties are best treated within the context of a small group where problems can be clarified, solutions generated, and plans for change implemented (Rose, 1977). Given that patients diagnosed with somatization disorder tend to have significant interpersonal difficulties (Zoccolillo &

Cloninger, 1986), group treatment may be the ideal setting for enhancing their social functioning. As an example, the role-playing component of assertiveness training, while sometimes awkward in individual therapy, is easily implemented in a group setting and actually is facilitated by the availability of group members who can assume various roles in the training while the therapist serves as a coach or director.

Group treatment reinforces and expands upon the cognitive, behavioral, and experiential methods addressed in individual treatment and encourages the development of interpersonal skills. The group, being a kind of transitional environment between individual therapy and the real world, helps patients transfer their new cognitive, emotional, and behavioral skills to everyday life. Each group session includes a "skill application" component during which patients discuss their experiences using cognitive, behavioral, and affective skills in their daily lives. The remainder of each group session is devoted to helping patients identify and express their thoughts and feelings to the group. This portion of the group sessions provides patients opportunities through role playing and other experiential exercises to develop greater awareness of, comfort with, and perspective on their thoughts and feelings. Although the focus of the group treatment is not entirely upon contemporaneous interactions among group members or upon group process, some element of interaction among group members is always present and is examined and used for its capacity to help patients identify and share thoughts and feelings. Group members give and receive feedback, often interpreted or facilitated by the group therapist. Patients respond to and are encouraged to explore and express their responses to individuals whose difficulties are similar to their own. In the group, patients receive the reactions of people they rarely encounter, peers whose personal experiences of suffering give their views a kind of credibility that the views of family members and healthcare professionals may not possess.

The rationale for beginning our intervention with individual treatment is as follows. Despite the evidence for somatization disorder being a discrete disorder (Katon et al., 1991), patients with somatization disorder may be highly heterogeneous in their specific somatic complaints, maladaptive behaviors, and dysfunctional beliefs (Bass & Murphy, 1991; Kirmayer, Robbins, & Paris, 1994; Smith et al., 1986a). Each patient also may present a singular pattern of comorbid disorders. Initiating treatment with individual sessions allows for individualization of treatment. Also, individual treatment is a preferable context for establishing a strong therapeutic alliance and facilitating a patient's commitment to therapy. Many patients with somatization, we have found, express pessimism about whether their disabilities are being regarded as real and serious and are being diligently and systematically addressed in treatment. They also are pessimistic regarding the capacity of a "talk therapy" to ameliorate their somatic symptoms (Kirmayer & Robbins, 1996; Lipowski, 1988). These various forms of pessimism are most readily confronted and dispelled in individual treatment, especially after some improvements in functioning and discomfort have occurred.

CONCLUSION AND FUTURE DIRECTIONS

Given the enormous costs of somatization disorder and its related syndromes to both patients and the healthcare system, there is a pressing need for effective treatments. The preceding paragraphs complete the presentation of the clinical description and rationale for our treatment. Our approach is evolving, even at this writing, and the future may bring additional exciting developments. Combining the tried and true methods of CBT with a focus on affect and experiential therapeutic techniques has seemed to some a dubious endeavor. Our own sense is that the experiential focus supplies what was missing in CBT; when the synthesis of the two approaches is applied by a skilled practitioner, there are great benefits for patients. Meanwhile, we have completed one randomized clinical trial in which the 10-session version of treatment demonstrated efficacy (Allen et al., 2006). This study is described in Appendix B. A second clinical trial (Escobar et al., 2006) conducted in a primary care setting has been completed, and we are in the midst of a trial testing the expanded ACBT.

Many years are required to test adequately the utility of any therapy. Time must pass before the initial enthusiasm of the innovators, the Hawthorne effects associated with the "latest scientific innovations," and the strong allegiances of early proponents fade and are no longer factors in enhancing efficacy and effectiveness. Time will tell.

Overview of Appendices

- *Appendix A. Ten-Session Treatment Manual*

  Appendix A provides a session-by-session outline of the treatment.

- *Appendix B. Clinical Trial Assessing the Efficacy of Affective Cognitive-Behavioral Therapy (ACBT)*

  Appendix B describes the first clinical trial assessing the efficacy of our 10-session ACBT for somatization disorder.

- *Appendix C. Severity of Somatic Symptoms Scale*

  Appendix C is a self-report inventory assessing the severity of somatic symptoms that are common in somatization syndromes. Total scores over 40 are indicative of at least moderate levels of physical discomfort.

- *Appendix D. Somatic Symptom Questionnaire*

  Appendix D is a self-report questionnaire designed to assess for the presence of somatization syndromes. Total scores over 5 are indicative of at least moderate somatization.

- *Appendix E. Instructions for Abbreviated Progressive Muscle Relaxation*

  Appendix E provides systematic instructions for the clinician to administer PMR. These instructions can be given to the patient to facilitate home practice of PMR.

- *Appendix F. Examining Thoughts*

  Appendix F provides a list of questions patients can use for examining their cognitions.

Ten-Session Treatment Manual

What follows is a 10-session version of our treatment. The treatment described in this appendix is, for reasons of practical necessity, succinct and highly structured. The 10-session treatment, comprising relaxation training, behavior modification, emotional awareness, cognitive restructuring, and interpersonal skills training, is an abbreviated subset of the full range of interventions that we employ with patients with somatization. It is conceptualized within a broad-spectrum cognitive-behavioral model, with special emphasis on the modification of illness behavior and the cognitions related to it.

The treatment manual presented herein is *not* intended to be a stand-alone or turn-key psychoeducational device that could be effectively employed by a healthcare worker who did not possess a background in the methods of psychotherapy employed, receive training in the application of methods, or have concurrent supervision. It was created to be the blueprint for a randomized clinical trial that would allow the empirical evaluation of a brief, standardized psychosocial intervention for somatization disorder. The use of the resulting 10-session treatment is justified by the cost-effectiveness considerations that are ubiquitous in the contemporary healthcare landscape and also warranted by the results of empirical research (Allen et al., 2006; Escobar et al., 2006), but we nevertheless view the brief treatment as an abridged version of a more comprehensive form of treatment that may be required to produce clinically meaningful and durable results with somatization patients. Chapters 5 through 9 describe the methods used in the 10-session treatment package as well as those additional methods employed in longer-term work with this population. This appendix details specific, session-by-session procedures followed by our therapists in the studies examining the efficacy of the 10-session version of our treatment (Allen et al., 2006; Escobar et al., 2006).

SESSION 1

In the first session the therapist has five aims: (1) to begin to establish rapport with the patient, (2) to provide an overview of the treatment and its rationale, (3) to review the patient's physical symptoms in the context(s) in which they occur, (4) to introduce the symptom-monitoring forms, (5) and to teach diaphragmatic breathing. The therapist should make every effort to accomplish all of these goals within 75–90 minutes. (Subsequent sessions are expected to last 60 minutes.) If necessary because of time constraints, the therapist can refrain from teaching diaphragmatic breathing until Session 2.

Establishing Rapport

As discussed earlier, engaging somatization patients in therapy is crucial. If the therapist senses that the patient has "one foot out the door" during the first session, the therapist may need to "sell" both the treatment and the therapist to the patient. If selling the treatment is necessary, the therapist should attempt a soft selling of it. That is, the therapist first needs to listen empathically as the patient describes his or her physical discomfort and emotional distress about living with such discomfort. Second, the therapist should acknowledge the patient's discomfort and distress as well as the patient's efforts to cope with the symptoms. Third, the therapist describes the treatment and its rationale without contradicting the patient's understanding of his or her symptoms.

Treatment Rationale

1. Discuss the physiological consequences of acute stress and chronic stress.
2. Describe the ways in which stress exacerbates physical symptoms.
3. Point out that chronic physical symptoms can become stressors in themselves.
4. Propose that reducing stress may improve physical discomfort.
5. Ask the patient to illustrate the ways in which stress affects his or her health.

Treatment Overview

1. Explain that treatment will consist of 10 sessions, one per week.
2. Describe the treatment as a skill-focused intervention.
3. Explain that a mastery of cognitive and behavioral skills requires practice between sessions and after treatment ends.
4. Clarify that treatment is a collaboration between patient and therapist.

Reviewing Target Symptoms

1. Review the patient's current physical complaints and the discomfort and impairment caused by each.

2. Identify the onset of each symptom.
3. Discuss previous treatment the patient has undergone for each symptom.
4. Identify the antecedents and consequences of each symptom.
5. Ask for the patient's hypotheses about the causes of the symptoms.
6. Discuss the patient's thoughts and feelings about the symptoms.

Introducing Symptom-Monitoring Forms

1. Provide a rationale for completing the symptom-monitoring forms.
2. Complete in session a monitoring form for an occasion within the previous 24 hours when the patient experienced a noteworthy elevation in physical discomfort as well as a time when he or she experienced relatively mild discomfort.

Teaching Diaphragmatic Breathing

1. Provide a rationale for breathing diaphragmatically.
2. Begin training in diaphragmatic breathing.

Homework

1. Complete a symptom-monitoring form each day.
2. Practice diaphragmatic breathing twice daily for 15-minute intervals.

SESSION 2

The goals of Session 2 are to discuss the patient's response to the initial session, review homework (symptom-monitoring forms and diaphragmatic breathing), assess the patient's activity level, and encourage an increase in activity (if appropriate) and/or activity pacing (if appropriate).

Reactions to Initial Session

1. Inquire into the patient's reactions to commencing a psychosocial treatment.
2. Review the treatment rationale and the patient's reaction to it.

Reviewing Symptom-Monitoring Forms

1. Discuss the patient's reactions to completing monitoring forms.
2. Validate and interpret as normative the patient's frustrations and difficulties completing the monitoring forms.
3. Review the rationale for completing monitoring forms.
4. If necessary, discuss the obstacles that interfered with completing the forms.

5. If necessary, problem-solve about completing the forms during the next week.
6. Review, in detail, two or three of the patient's entries on the forms.
7. Discuss patterns the patient has observed as a consequence of completing the forms this week (e.g., his or her symptoms are worse in the evenings or after arguments).
8. Provide additional training on completing the forms properly (e.g., correctly identifying physical symptoms, thoughts, and emotions).

Reviewing Diaphragmatic Breathing

1. Review the rationale for diaphragmatic breathing.
2. Discuss the patient's practice of breathing (when, where, for what duration, how often practice occurred?).
3. Inquire into the patient's emotional and physical reactions during diaphragmatic breathing.
4. If necessary, discuss the obstacles that interfered with engaging in relaxation.
5. If necessary, problem-solve about engaging in relaxation during the next week.
6. Ask the patient to breathe diaphragmatically in session for 2–3 minutes.
7. Discuss the patient's experience while breathing diaphragmatically in session.
8. Discuss the therapist's observations of the patient's breathing in session.

Activity Assessment and Change

1. Conduct a detailed behavioral assessment. How does the patient spend his or her time?
2. Ask how the patient's physical symptoms have affected his or her activities.
3. Discuss the rationale for making behavioral changes.
4. Collaborate with the patient in identifying long-term and short-term behavioral goals for exercise as well as goals for meaningful and pleasurable activities.
5. Discuss activity pacing (e.g., making changes gradually, taking breaks).
6. Collaborate with the patient to make a specific activity plan for the next week.

Homework

1. Practice diaphragmatic breathing twice daily for 15-minute intervals.
2. Continue completing the symptom-monitoring forms daily.
3. Carry out the new activity plan, including activity pacing.

SESSION 3 (WITH SPOUSE/SIGNIFICANT OTHER)

The primary goal of Session 3 is to increase the likelihood that the patient's significant other will support and not undermine treatment. By meeting with the significant other, the therapist may learn additional information about the patient's symptoms and functioning. Finally, if time permits in this session or in future conjoint sessions, the therapist attempts to aid the couple in making small changes in their behavior and/or interaction.

Introduction to Significant Other

1. Discuss the rationale for stress-management treatment.
2. Ask the significant other for his or her observations regarding the impact of stress on the patient's symptoms.

Reviewing Diaphragmatic Breathing

1. Review the rationale for diaphragmatic breathing.
2. Practice breathing diaphragmatically with the patient (and significant other, if willing).
3. Discuss the patient's experience with breathing diaphragmatically this week.

Reviewing Behavioral Assignment

1. Review the rationale for increasing and pacing activities.
2. Review the patient's behavioral homework assignment (when, where, for what duration, how often activity occurred?).
3. Discuss the patient's emotional and physical reactions while carrying out the behavioral homework assignment.

Planning Pleasurable Couple Activities

1. Discuss the rationale for increasing pleasurable couple activities.
2. Conduct an assessment of the couple's current and past joint activities.
3. Collaborate with the patient and significant other to create a list of potential pleasurable activities.
4. Encourage the couple to make a specific couple activity plan for the upcoming month.

Discussing Couple's Communication about Symptoms (if time permits)

(Note: Time limitations usually result in postponing discussion of the couple's communication until the second conjoint session. If the couple begins treatment already engaged in pleasurable couple's activities, however, the therapist will have time to begin the couple's communication discussion in the first conjoint session.)

1. Review a recent interaction between the patient and significant other about the patient's symptoms.
2. Identify and discuss with the couple the communication tendencies elicited from the above discussion (see examples listed in Chapter 8).
3. Ask the couple to role-play alternative communication styles in session.
4. Plan "communication experiments" for the couple to carry out at home.

Homework

1. Practice diaphragmatic breathing twice daily for 15-minute intervals.
2. Continue completing the symptom-monitoring forms daily.
3. Carry out the new activity plan, including activity pacing.
4. Carry out conjoint pleasurable activities.
5. Attempt communication experiments, if discussed in session.

SESSION 4

Incorporating Breathing into Daily Life

1. Discuss the patient's diaphragmatic breathing over the past week.
2. Review the rationale for breathing diaphragmatically during everyday activities.
3. Have the patient attempt to breathe diaphragmatically throughout today's session.
4. Check in with the patient about his or her breathing every 5–10 minutes during the session.
5. At end of session, review the patient's experience attending to his or her breathing during the session.
6. Plan specific situations in which the patient will combine diaphragmatic breathing with other activities.

Reviewing Other Homework

1. Briefly discuss the patient's reactions to the couple's session.
2. Discuss the patient's individual activity assignment and his or her progress toward the short-term and long-term behavioral goals identified in Session 2.
3. Review two of the patient's entries on the symptom-monitoring forms.

Sleep Hygiene and Stimulus Control Techniques

1. Conduct a sleep assessment. (If the patient appears to have no difficulty sleeping, the therapist omits the remainder of the sleep section. If not, the therapist continues.)

2. Discuss the rationale for sleep hygiene and stimulus control techniques.
3. Collaborate with the patient to develop a plan for changing bedtime and bedroom activities to enhance sleep.
4. Encourage the patient to use diaphragmatic breathing to relax while lying in bed at night.

Distraction

1. Discuss the rationale for distraction.
2. Collaborate with the patient to create a list of potentially distracting activities.
3. Help the patient plan specific distraction experiments for homework.

Homework

1. Practice diaphragmatic breathing twice daily for 15 minutes when sitting quietly.
2. Breathe diaphragmatically during other activities (e.g., watching TV, talking on the phone, using the computer).
3. Continue completing the symptom-monitoring forms daily.
4. Carry out the activity plan, including activity pacing.
5. Use sleep hygiene and stimulus control techniques as discussed above.
6. Use distraction experiments three to four times this week.

SESSION 5

Reviewing Homework

1. Discuss the patient's experience using diaphragmatic breathing during daily activities.
2. Discuss the patient's individual activity assignment and his or her progress toward the short-term and long-term behavioral goals identified in Session 2.
3. Discuss the patient's experience using sleep hygiene and stimulus control techniques, if appropriate.
4. Discuss the patient's experience using distraction.
5. Review one entry on the symptom-monitoring forms.

Cognitive Restructuring

1. Discuss the rationale for cognitive restructuring, labeled for patients as "examining thoughts more deeply."
2. Select a thought from the patient's symptom-monitoring forms to be challenged. The therapist attempts to select a thought that this patient has articulated repeatedly.

3. Encourage the patient to read aloud and answer questions from the Examining Thoughts handout (Appendix F) as a means of challenging thoughts.
4. If time permits, guide the patient in challenging (with the Examining Thoughts handout) a second thought from the patient's symptom-monitoring forms.

Homework

1. Practice diaphragmatic breathing twice daily for 15 minutes when sitting quietly.
2. Breathe diaphragmatically during other activities (e.g., watching TV, talking on the phone, using the computer).
3. Continue completing the symptom-monitoring forms.
4. Examine thoughts more deeply (i.e., challenge cognitions).
5. Continue carrying out the activity plan and activity pacing.
6. Continue using sleep hygiene and stimulus control techniques, if appropriate.
7. Continue using distraction, if appropriate.

SESSION 6

Reviewing Homework

1. Discuss the patient's experience using diaphragmatic breathing during daily activities.
2. Discuss the patient's activity homework.
3. Discuss the patient's experience using sleep hygiene and stimulus control techniques, if appropriate.
4. Discuss the patient's experience using distraction, if appropriate.

Reviewing Cognitive Restructuring

1. Discuss the patient's experience examining thoughts deeply (i.e., cognitive restructuring).
2. Review each thought the patient examined for homework.

Teaching Abbreviated Progressive Muscle Relaxation (PMR)

1. Discuss the rationale for PMR.
2. Guide the patient through PMR (Appendix E).

Homework

1. Practice PMR in quiet settings twice daily.
2. Breathe diaphragmatically during other activities (e.g., watching TV, talking the on phone, using the computer).

3. Continue completing the symptom-monitoring forms.
4. Examine thoughts more deeply (i.e., challenge cognitions).
5. Continue carrying out the activity plan and activity pacing.
6. Continue using sleep hygiene and stimulus control techniques, if appropriate.
7. Continue using distraction, if appropriate.

SESSION 7 (WITH SIGNIFICANT OTHER)

Reviewing Homework

1. Discuss the patient's experience using PMR.
2. Discuss the patient's use of diaphragmatic breathing during daily activities.
3. Discuss the patient's individual activity assignment and progress toward his or her behavioral goals.
4. Discuss the patient's experience using sleep hygiene and stimulus control techniques, if appropriate.

(Note: Distraction and cognitive restructuring are not reviewed in conjoint sessions.)

Reviewing Couple's Pleasurable Activities

1. Review the rationale for engaging in couple's pleasurable activities.
2. Discuss the couple's experience carrying out pleasurable activities discussed in Session 3.
3. Assist the couple in planning future joint activities.

Reviewing Couple's Communication

1. Review the rationale for improving communication between patient and significant other.
2. Discuss the couple's communication skills and problems.
3. Ask the couple to role-play alternative communication styles in session.
4. Plan communication experiments for the couple to carry out at home.

(It is important to acknowledge to the significant other and patient that there are too few sessions to make substantial changes in the couple's behavior. Couple therapy may be discussed as a future option, if indicated.)

Homework

1. Use PMR and/or diaphragmatic breathing in quiet settings and during other activities.
2. Attempt communication experiments, if discussed in session.

3. Continue carrying out the activity plans (individual's and couple's).
4. Continue completing the symptom-monitoring forms.
5. Continue using sleep hygiene and stimulus control techniques, if appropriate.

SESSION 8

Reviewing Homework

1. Discuss the patient's experience using PMR and diaphragmatic breathing.
2. Discuss the individual and couple activity assignments.
3. Discuss the patient's experience with sleep hygiene and stimulus control techniques, if appropriate.
4. Discuss the patient's experience using distraction, if appropriate.
5. Discuss one or two thoughts the patient examined (i.e., challenged) over the past 2 weeks.

Discussing the Sick Role

1. Ask the patient to think about other people he or she has known well who have been ill.
2. Ask about the advantages and disadvantages of illness for those people.
3. Ask the patient to consider the impact of illness on his or her past and current life (including both the advantages and disadvantages of the symptoms for the patient).

Teaching Assertiveness Skills

1. Discuss the rationale for and definition of assertiveness.
2. Introduce the use of "I" statements to express one's thoughts and feelings.
3. Assist the patient in selecting a situation in which he or she acted unassertively in the past.
4. Role-play with the patient to demonstrate more assertive responses in this situation.
5. Role-play with the patient to demonstrate more assertive responses in one or two other situations, time permitting.
6. Assist the patient in planning assertiveness experiments to conduct over the next week.

Homework

1. Use PMR and/or diaphragmatic breathing in quiet settings and during other activities.
2. Continue carrying out the activity plan.
3. Continue completing the symptom-monitoring forms.

4. Continue examining thoughts more deeply (i.e., restructuring cognitions).
5. Continue using sleep hygiene and stimulus control techniques, if appropriate.
6. Continue using distraction, if appropriate.
7. Conduct the assertiveness assignment discussed in session.

SESSION 9

Reviewing Homework

1. Discuss the patient's experience using PMR and diaphragmatic breathing.
2. Discuss the individual activity assignments and progress toward the patient's short-term and long-term behavioral goals.
3. Discuss the patient's experience with sleep hygiene and stimulus control techniques, if appropriate.
4. Discuss the patient's experience using distraction, if appropriate.
5. Discuss one or two thoughts the patient examined (i.e., challenged) over the past 2 weeks.

Reviewing Assertiveness

1. Discuss the patient's experience attempting the assertiveness assignment.
2. Conduct additional training in assertiveness, usually with multiple role plays.
3. Collaborate with the patient in planning future assertive actions.

Homework

1. Use PMR and/or diaphragmatic breathing in quiet settings and during other activities.
2. Continue carrying out the individual activity plan.
3. Continue examining thoughts more deeply (i.e., challenging cognitions).
4. Continue using sleep hygiene and stimulus control techniques, if appropriate.
5. Continue using distraction, if appropriate.
6. Conduct the assertiveness assignment discussed in session.

SESSION 10 (WITH SIGNIFICANT OTHER, IF POSSIBLE)

Reviewing Homework

1. Discuss the patient's experience using PMR and diaphragmatic breathing.
2. Discuss the individual and couple activity assignments and future behavioral goals.

3. Discuss the patient's experience with sleep hygiene and stimulus control techniques, if appropriate.
4. Discuss the couple's communication assignment.

Reviewing Stress-Management Skills

1. Review the patient's ongoing use of each stress-management technique discussed during the course of treatment (i.e., diaphragmatic breathing, PMR, increasing activities alone and with significant other, increasing exercise, pacing activities, distraction, challenging thoughts, sleep hygiene, communication skills with significant other, and assertiveness).
2. Discuss the warning signs that the patient may need help from others (e.g., friends, family, healthcare providers) in managing stress.
3. Discuss the possibility of additional or booster treatment.

Discussing Termination

1. Discuss patient's feelings about terminating.
2. Bid farewell.

Clinical Trial Assessing the Efficacy of Affective Cognitive-Behavioral Therapy

What follows is an abbreviated, reader-friendly report of an elaborate clinical trial. We have omitted some variables studied and analyses conducted.

We conducted a randomized, controlled treatment trial in which 84 patients diagnosed with full somatization disorder received one of two treatments: either (1) the control intervention, augmented standard medical care, or (2) our 10-session affective cognitive-behavioral therapy (ACBT) combined with augmented standard medical care. In both treatment conditions, standard medical care was augmented by sending to patients' primary care physicians the psychiatric consultation letter employed by Smith and colleagues (1986b) with minor modifications to make it applicable to our research environment. The study thus employed an additive design, in which a treatment to be tested is added to another treatment to determine whether the treatment added produces an incremental improvement over the first treatment.

Participants, recruited from medical clinics and community advertisements, were evaluated during screening and baseline interviews. Afterward, they were randomly assigned to one of the two treatment conditions. Patients were reassessed at a posttreatment assessment, which occurred 3 months after baseline, and at two separate follow-up evaluations, 6 months and 12 months following the posttreatment assessment (i.e., 9 and 15 months after baseline). By augmenting both the control and experimental patients' standard medical care, the present study established a relatively conservative test of the treatment's efficacy, in that significant findings would be obtained only if the psychosocial treatment produced improvements over and above those resulting from the psychiatric consultation letter intervention, an efficacious intervention in previous research (Rost et al., 1994; Smith et al., 1986b, 1995).

METHODS

Participants

Eighty-four men and women, aged 18–70 years and meeting DSM-IV criteria for somatization disorder, were included in the study. Potential participants were excluded on the following bases: (1) having a serious and unstable medical condition, (2) having a history of psychotic disorder or organic brain syndrome, or (3) having a current alcohol or substance use disorder. Patients meeting DSM-IV criteria for affective disorders, anxiety disorders, or eating disorders comorbid with somatization disorder were included unless patients indicated their comorbid psychiatric disorder(s) caused greater distress or functional impairment than did the physical discomfort resulting from their unexplained symptoms. Use of concurrent medication was permitted, as long as it had been stabilized for 2 months prior to study entry. Also, participants were requested not to alter their medication regimens during the study.

Treatments

Affective Cognitive-Behavioral Therapy for Somatization Disorder

The treatment was 10 weekly 60-minute sessions of our manualized intervention, outlined in Appendix A. When available, the patient's significant other/partner was invited to participate in as many as three of the 10 treatment sessions.

Augmented Standard Medical Care

All 84 study participants were allowed to receive medical treatment as needed for their physical distress throughout the study. The medical treatment is referred to as "augmented standard medical care" (ASMC) because standard medical care was supplemented by the psychiatric consultation intervention that has shown efficacy in previous research (Rost et al., 1994; Smith et al., 1986b, 1995). This letter was sent to all patients' primary physicians. It stated that the patient met DSM-IV criteria for a diagnosis of somatization disorder and provided the following recommendations for treatment:

1. Schedule regular appointments every 4–6 weeks with the patient.
2. At each visit, conduct a physical examination in the organ system or body part relevant to the presenting complaint.
3. Avoid unnecessary diagnostic procedures, invasive treatments, and hospitalizations.
4. Avoid making disparaging statements such as "Your symptoms are all in your head."

Therapists and Training

Four therapists, either masters- or doctoral-level psychologists experienced in cognitive-behavioral therapy, conducted the treatment. All therapists participated in didactic and clinical training with at least one of the authors prior to treating a study participant. The training included a detailed review and explanation of the treatment manual and participation as a cotherapist in treating nonstudy patients. Also, therapists received weekly individual supervision by one of us based on reviewing audiotaped treatment sessions.

Assessments

Participants were evaluated at the screening and baseline appointments as well as 3 months after baseline (posttreatment), 6 months after posttreatment, and 12 months after posttreatment. The interviewers conducting all assessments were blind to the participants' treatment condition.

At the screening appointment, eligibility for the study was determined by reviewing patients' medical and psychiatric histories. First, patients described their medical histories. Afterward, the Structured Clinical Interview for DSM-IV Axis I Disorders (SCID-I; First et al., 1997) was administered to confirm the diagnosis and to ascertain psychiatric history. The physician most central in the treatment of the patient's unexplained physical symptoms (usually the patient's primary care physician or rheumatologist) was contacted by telephone to confirm physical diagnoses.

For eligible participants there were four assessments in addition to the screening appointment. At each of the other four assessment appointments (baseline, posttreatment, 6 months following posttreatment, and 12 months following posttreatment) identical assessment batteries were administered that provided the data for evaluating the treatment's efficacy. At each of these appointments, the various measures of somatic symptoms and physical functioning were administered as described below.

The study's primary outcome measure was an independent evaluator's judgment of the severity of somatization, measured by the Clinical Global Impression Scale for Somatization Disorder (CGI-SD). The CGI-SD yields a composite symptom severity rating made by a trained rater after questioning the patient about the current frequency of, intensity of, and impairment caused by the 33 somatic symptoms that are assessed in assigning a DSM-IV diagnosis of somatization disorder. At baseline, the CGI-SD consists of one item, a severity item. At the other three assessment sessions, the CGI-SD consists of two items, a severity and an improvement item. Severity is rated on a 7-point Likert-type scale ranging from 1 (no somatization) to 7 (very severe, among the most extreme cases of somatization). Improvement is rated on another 7-point Likert-type scale ranging from 1 (very much improved) to 7 (very much worse). Treatment response was defined as a rating of a 1 (very much improved) or a 2 (much improved) on the CGI-SD Improvement scale.

The physical functioning subscale of the Medical Outcomes Study 36-Item Short Form Health Survey (MOS SF-36; Ware & Sherbourne, 1992) was administered at each of the four assessment sessions to measure impairment in physical activities, such as in climbing stairs, kneeling, or walking various distances. Chapter 4 provides additional information about the MOS SF-36.

Somatic symptoms were measured by self-reports recorded in daily symptom diaries and by the Severity of Somatic Symptoms scale. In the symptom diaries, at the end of each day, patients recorded the maximum severity of their physical symptoms on that day. Ratings were made on 6-point Likert-type items (0 = no physical discomfort to 5 = extreme physical discomfort). Mean maximum discomfort scores were computed from subjects' ratings for the 7 consecutive days immediately prior to each of the assessment sessions (baseline, posttreatment, 6 months following posttreatment, and 12 months following posttreatment). Also, at these four assessment sessions, patients completed a self-report inventory of somatization symptoms, the Severity of Somatic Symptoms scale (SSS). The SSS requires subjects to rate on 8-point Likert-type items the degree to which they were troubled, over the previous month, by each of 40 somatization symptoms. (See Chapter 4 for a description of the symptom diaries and the SSS.)

Healthcare utilization was assessed by examining participants' medical records for the 12-month interval prior to baseline and for the 15-month interval following baseline. At the baseline appointment, patients were asked to sign a consent form allowing the research team to obtain information from all insurance carriers and healthcare providers (physicians/nonphysicians, physical/mental health providers, inpatient/outpatient facilities) they had used over the previous 12 months. At each assessment point, participants were asked to review and revise their list of insurers and providers to include all new providers and/or insurers. A list of all services and costs of services provided during the pretreatment year and the 15 months of the study was requested from both insurance companies and providers. These requests were made multiple times, when necessary, to obtain the information.

RESULTS

Treatment Groups at Baseline

There were no significant differences in baseline characteristics between the two treatment groups (Table B.1). The majority of participants were middle-aged women who had suffered from unexplained physical symptoms for an average of 25 years.

An examination of participants' referral sources revealed that 59 participants (70.2%) were recruited from healthcare practitioners (i.e., physician referrals) and 25 (29.8%) were recruited from public advertisements (self-referrals). No demographic nor clinical differences were observed between physician referrals and self-referrals. The two treatment conditions were not different in the proportion of physician referrals versus self-referrals.

Attrition

Attrition rates were low throughout the study. Only seven patients (8.3%) withdrew before the posttreatment assessment, four from the ACBT and three

TABLE B.1. Baseline Characteristics of the Participants

	ACBT + ASMC (*n* = 43)	ASMC (*n* = 41)	*p*
Age, mean (*SD*), years	45.47 (8.45)	47.85 (10.99)	.27
Female, No. (%)	36 (83.72)	39 (95.12)	.09
Race/Ethnicity, No. (%)			
White	36 (83.72)	33 (80.49)	
African American	1 (2.33)	2 (4.88)	.94
Hispanic	5 (11.63)	5 (12.20)	
Other	1 (2.33)	1 (2.44)	
Education, No. (%)			
Graduate degree	6 (13.95)	7 (17.07)	
College degree	16 (37.21)	9 (21.95)	
Some college	9 (20.93)	14 (34.15)	.46
High school degree	11 (25.58)	9 (21.95)	
Some high school	1 (2.33)	2 (4.88)	
Married, No. (%)	23 (53.49)	22 (53.66)	.99
Employed, No. (%)	23 (53.49)	23 (56.10)	.81
Receiving disability, No. (%)	9 (20.93)	7 (17.07)	.65
Hollingshead SES, mean (*SD*)	47.70 (9.65)	45.49 (9.59)	.30
Current comorbid DSM-IV Axis I disorder, No. (%)	30 (69.77)	24 (58.54)	.28
Duration of symptoms, mean (*SD*), years	24.95 (11.54)	25.00 (15.12)	.99
Referred by physician, No. (%)	32 (74.42)	27 (65.85)	.39

Note. ACBT, affective cognitive-behavioral therapy; ASMC, standard medical care augmented by a psychiatric consultation letter; Hollingshead SES, Hollingshead Socioeconomic Status scale score; DSM-IV, *Diagnostic and Statistical Manual of Mental Disorders*, fourth edition.

from the control condition. A total of 11 participants failed to complete the 6-month follow-up; 12 participants were unavailable for the 12-month follow-up assessment. The two treatment conditions did not differ from each other in the number of participants who failed to attend any of the posttreatment or follow-up sessions. Dropouts were not significantly different from treatment completers on any clinical measure.

Treatment Outcome

Mixed-model repeated-measures analysis of variance (ANOVA) on the intent-to-treat sample was the primary analytic approach with parametric variables. For the primary outcome measure, CGI-SD severity, this analysis resulted in statistically significant effects for treatment condition ($F_{1,82} = 5.86$, $p = .02$), for time ($F_{3,82} = 29.96$, $p < .001$), and for the treatment-by-time inter-action ($F_{3,82} = 11.00$, $p < .001$). Planned contrasts revealed significantly greater reductions in CGI-SD severity scores for ACBT participants than for control participants between baseline and each of the follow-up evaluations: posttreatment ($F_{1,82} = 16.33$, $p < .001$), 6 months posttreatment ($F_{1,82} = 27.08$, $p < .001$), and 12 months posttreatment ($F_{1,82} = 22.55$, $p < .001$). The effect sizes for the treatment effect on CGI-SD severity were $d = 0.60$ at post-treatment, $d = 0.95$ at 6 months posttreatment, and $d = 0.92$ at 12 months posttreatment.

All parametric secondary endpoints were analyzed with same mixed-model repeated-measures ANOVA described above. On self-reported physi-cal functioning (MOS SF-36) this analysis resulted in significant effects for time ($F_{3,82} = 8.70$, $p < .001$) and for the treatment-by-time interaction ($F_{3,82} = 3.66$, $p = .02$). Planned contrasts showed that ACBT participants' scores improved significantly more than control participants' scores between base-line and each follow-up assessment: posttreatment ($F_{1,82} = 9.82$, $p = .002$), 6 months posttreatment ($F_{1,82} = 6.19$, $p = .01$), and 12 months posttreatment ($F_{1,82} = 6.74$, $p = .01$). The effect sizes for the treatment effect on the MOS SF-36 were $d = 0.22$ at posttreatment, $d = 0.30$ at 6 months posttreatment, and $d = 0.32$ at 12 months posttreatment. For the symptom diary, significant effects were obtained for time ($F_{3,82} = 6.67$, $p < .001$) as well as for the treatment-by-time interaction ($F_{3,82} = 6.89$, $p < .001$). Planned contrasts revealed greater decreases in somatic symptom severity, recorded in daily diaries, for ACBT than for control participants at each follow-up assessment: posttreatment ($F_{1,82} = 8.18$, $p = .008$), 6 months posttreatment ($F_{1,82} = 19.80$, $p < .001$), and 12 months posttreatment ($F_{1,82} = 9.92$, $p = .002$). The effect sizes for the treatment effect on the symptom diary were $d = 0.66$ at posttreatment, $d = 0.91$ at 6 months posttreatment, and $d = 0.75$ at 12 months posttreatment. Similarly, for the Severity of Somatic Symptoms (SSS) Scale, there was a significant effect for time ($F_{3,82} = 15.73$, $p < .001$) and for the treatment-by-time interaction ($F_{3,82} = 3.97$, $p = .01$). Planned contrasts on the SSS showed greater reductions in retrospectively recorded somatic symptom severity at each follow-up assess-ment in favor of ACBT: posttreatment ($F_{1,82} = 9.01$, $p = .003$), 6 months posttreatment ($F_{1,82} = 9.70$, $p = .002$), and 12 months posttreatment ($F_{1,82} = 8.01$, $p = .005$). The effect sizes for the treatment effect on SSS were $d = 0.35$ at posttreatment, $d = 0.50$ at 6 months posttreatment, and $d = 0.34$ at 12 months posttreatment.

Responder analyses conducted on the CGI-SD improvement scale re-vealed a significantly greater proportion of ACBT participants were rated by an independent evaluator as "much improved" or "very much improved" at each of the assessments following treatment (all three Fisher's exact test $ps < .001$) as compared with control participants (Figure B.1).

Complete healthcare records were obtained for 56 (67.5%) of the study sample. There were no differences in baseline demographic or clinical charac-teristics between participants for whom complete healthcare records were

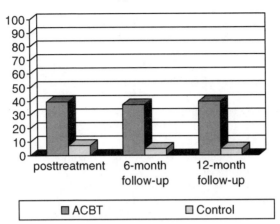

FIGURE B.1. Percent of participants rated as "much improved" or "very much improved" on the Clinical Global Impression Improvement Scale (CGI-I).

obtained and those for whom healthcare records were either unavailable or incomplete. Among participants with complete healthcare records, there were no differences on baseline demographic or clinical measures between participants in the ACBT and control conditions. Exploratory nonparametric tests were performed on the other measures of healthcare utilization. Mann–Whitney tests revealed a greater reduction in total costs ($Z = 2.45$, $p = .01$) for ACBT participants than for control participants. Between-group differences in favor of ACBT approached significance on the number of physician visits ($Z = 1.84$, $p = .07$). The two groups did not differ on the number of diagnostic procedures conducted after the treatment phase of the study.

DISCUSSION

Our study is the first randomized clinical trial that has successfully treated patients with full somatization disorder as defined by DSM-IV. We found statistically significant effects for our treatment on several measures of symptom severity and physical functioning. On the CGI-SD, the magnitude of an effect rated as clinically meaningful was more frequently observed in the ACBT group than in the control group.

This report of the clinical trial is preliminary and more data remain to be analyzed. The findings are consistent with those of another study at our center (Escobar et al., 2006) that utilized our 10-session treatment in a primary care setting to treat successfully a sample of heterogeneous and, on average, less impaired patients with somatization.

FUTURE DIRECTIONS

Given the success of the brief, manualized ACBT in two different investigations, there is indication that this treatment should be disseminated and subjected to further tests of efficacy and effectiveness. Comparisons between our brief treatment and other interventions (e.g., conventional psychotherapy or pharmacotherapy) are obvious targets for future research. As discussed in Chapters 5 through 9, we have expanded the treatment. Our more comprehensive treatment is currently being evaluated in a clinical trial that is funded by the National Institute of Mental Health (No. R21 MH066831).

Severity of Somatic Symptoms Scale

Circle the number corresponding to the amount of distress you have experienced from each of the following symptoms *over the past month*. If you have not experienced the symptom at all this month, please circle 0.

1. Abdominal or belly pain (not counting times when you were menstruating)

0	1	2	3	4	5	6	7
not at all							so much I could barely stand it

2. Back pain

0	1	2	3	4	5	6	7
not at all							so much I could barely stand it

3. Pains in your joints (knees, elbows, etc.)

0	1	2	3	4	5	6	7
not at all							so much I could barely stand it

4. Pains in your arms or legs other than joint pains

0	1	2	3	4	5	6	7
not at all							so much I could barely stand it

(continued)

5. Chest pains

0	1	2	3	4	5	6	7
not at all							so much I could barely stand it

6. Headaches

0	1	2	3	4	5	6	7
not at all							so much I could barely stand it

7. Excessively painful menstrual periods

0	1	2	3	4	5	6	7
not at all							so much I could barely stand it

8. Pain when you urinated—that is, passed your water

0	1	2	3	4	5	6	7
not at all							so much I could barely stand it

9. Burning pain in your "private parts"

0	1	2	3	4	5	6	7
not at all							so much I could barely stand it

10. Any other pain, pain not described in questions 1–9 (describe: _____)

0	1	2	3	4	5	6	7
not at all							so much I could barely stand it

11. Vomiting

0	1	2	3	4	5	6	7
not at all							so much I could barely stand it

12. Nausea—that is, feeling sick to your stomach but not actually vomiting

0	1	2	3	4	5	6	7
not at all							so much I could barely stand it

(continued)

13. Loose bowels or diarrhea

0	1	2	3	4	5	6	7
not at all							so much I could barely stand it

14. Excessive gas or bloating of your stomach or abdomen

0	1	2	3	4	5	6	7
not at all							so much I could barely stand it

15. Inability to eat several kinds of foods because they made you ill

0	1	2	3	4	5	6	7
not at all							so much I could barely stand it

16. Loss of vision in one or both eyes to the extent that you couldn't see anything at all for a few seconds or more

0	1	2	3	4	5	6	7
not at all							so much I could barely stand it

17. Blurred vision for some period not due to needing glasses or changing glasses

0	1	2	3	4	5	6	7
not at all							so much I could barely stand it

18. Loss of hearing for a period of time

0	1	2	3	4	5	6	7
not at all							so much I could barely stand it

19. Trouble walking

0	1	2	3	4	5	6	7
not at all							so much I could barely stand it

(continued)

20. Loss of feeling in an arm or a leg (at times **other** than when it had just fallen asleep or become numb from being in one position too long)

0	1	2	3	4	5	6	7
not at all							so much I could barely stand it

21. Inability to move a part of your body for at least a few minutes

0	1	2	3	4	5	6	7
not at all							so much I could barely stand it

22. Loss of your voice for 30 minutes or more and inability to speak above a whisper

0	1	2	3	4	5	6	7
not at all							so much I could barely stand it

23. A seizure or convulsion causing you to become unconscious or causing your body to jerk uncontrollably

0	1	2	3	4	5	6	7
not at all							so much I could barely stand it

24. Fainting (or falling out) spells where you felt weak or dizzy and then passed out

0	1	2	3	4	5	6	7
not at all							so much I could barely stand it

25. Being unconscious for any other reason

0	1	2	3	4	5	6	7
not at all							so much I could barely stand it

26. A period of amnesia

0	1	2	3	4	5	6	7
not at all							so much I could barely stand it

(continued)

27. Double vision

0	1	2	3	4	5	6	7
not at all							so much I could barely stand it

28. Shortness of breath when you had not been exercising or exerting yourself

0	1	2	3	4	5	6	7
not at all							so much I could barely stand it

29. Your heart beating so hard that you could feel it pound in your chest

0	1	2	3	4	5	6	7
not at all							so much I could barely stand it

30. Dizziness

0	1	2	3	4	5	6	7
not at all							so much I could barely stand it

31. Periods of weakness, when you could not lift or move things you could normally lift or move

0	1	2	3	4	5	6	7
not at all							so much I could barely stand it

32. A lot of blotchiness or discoloration of the skin

0	1	2	3	4	5	6	7
not at all							so much I could barely stand it

33. A lot of trouble with a bad taste in your mouth or an excessively coated tongue

0	1	2	3	4	5	6	7
not at all							so much I could barely stand it

(continued)

34. Having to urinate so frequently that it caused you trouble

0	1	2	3	4	5	6	7
not at all							so much I could barely stand it

35. Unpleasant numbness or tingling sensations

0	1	2	3	4	5	6	7
not at all							so much I could barely stand it

36. The feeling of a lump in your throat that made it difficult to swallow

0	1	2	3	4	5	6	7
not at all							so much I could barely stand it

37. Irregular menstrual periods

0	1	2	3	4	5	6	7
not at all							so much I could barely stand it

38. Excessive bleeding with your menstrual periods

0	1	2	3	4	5	6	7
not at all							so much I could barely stand it

39. Inability to urinate when you felt like you had to urinate

0	1	2	3	4	5	6	7
not at all							so much I could barely stand it

40. Vomiting during pregnancy

0	1	2	3	4	5	6	7
not at all							so much I could barely stand it

Total Score (sum of items 1–40) _____

Somatic Symptom Questionnaire

We would like you to tell us about some physical symptoms people often experience. By marking "Yes" or "No" in the blanks after the following statements, indicate whether you have experienced the symptom described in the statement. If you have never experienced the symptom described in part A of the question, skip sections B–D of that item and go to the next numbered question. If you have experienced the symptom described in part A of the question, please answer parts B–D. If the symptom was entirely due to a physical illness or an accident, please indicate so in the space provided after the statement. Also, please indicate whether you consulted a doctor for this symptom. If you received a diagnosis as a result of the consultation, please write the diagnosis in the blank provided.

1. A) Have you ever had a lot of trouble with abdominal or belly pain (not counting times you were menstruating)? Yes _____ No _____
   B) If yes, was that symptom due to a physical illness or an accident? Yes _____ No _____
   C) Have you seen a doctor for that symptom? Yes _____ No _____
   D) If yes, what was the doctor's diagnosis? _____

2. A) Have you ever had a lot of trouble with back pain? Yes _____ No _____
   B) If yes, was that symptom due to a physical illness or an accident? Yes _____ No _____
   C) Have you seen a doctor for that symptom? Yes _____ No _____
   D) If yes, what was the doctor's diagnosis? _____

3. A) Have you ever had pains in your joints (knees, elbows, etc.)? Yes _____ No _____
   B) If yes, was that symptom due to a physical illness or an accident? Yes _____ No _____
   C) Have you seen a doctor for that symptom? Yes _____ No _____
   D) If yes, what was the doctor's diagnosis? _____

(continued)

4. A) Have you ever had pains in your arms or legs other than joint pains? Yes _____ No _____
    B) If yes, was that symptom due to a physical illness or an accident? Yes _____ No _____
    C) Have you seen a doctor for that symptom? Yes _____ No _____
    D) If yes, what was the doctor's diagnosis? _____

5. A) Have you ever had chest pains? Yes _____ No _____
    B) If yes, was that symptom due to a physical illness or an accident? Yes _____ No _____
    C) Have you seen a doctor for that symptom? Yes _____ No _____
    D) If yes, what was the doctor's diagnosis? _____

6. A) Have you ever had a lot of trouble with headaches? Yes _____ No _____
    B) If yes, was that symptom due to a physical illness or an accident? Yes _____ No _____
    C) Have you seen a doctor for that symptom? Yes _____ No _____
    D) If yes, what was the doctor's diagnosis? _____

7. A) Have you ever had a lot of trouble with excessively painful menstrual periods? Yes _____ No _____
    B) If yes, was that symptom due to a physical illness or an accident? Yes _____ No _____
    C) Have you seen a doctor for that symptom? Yes _____ No _____
    D) If yes, what was the doctor's diagnosis? _____

8. A) Have you ever had pain when you urinated—that is passed your water? Yes _____ No _____
    B) If yes, was that symptom due to a physical illness or an accident? Yes _____ No _____
    C) Have you seen a doctor for that symptom? Yes _____ No _____
    D) If yes, what was the doctor's diagnosis? _____

9. A) Has there ever been a time lasting 24 hours or longer when you were completely unable to urinate or had great difficulty urinating (other than after either childbirth or surgery)? Yes _____ No _____
    B) If yes, was that symptom due to a physical illness or an accident? Yes _____ No _____
    C) Have you seen a doctor for that symptom? Yes _____ No _____
    D) If yes, what was the doctor's diagnosis? _____

10. A) Have you ever had burning pain in your "private parts"? Yes _____ No _____
    B) If yes, was that symptom due to a physical illness or an accident? Yes _____ No _____

(continued)

C) Have you seen a doctor for that symptom? Yes _____ No _____

D) If yes, what was the doctor's diagnosis? _____

11. A) Have you ever had any other pain, pain not described in questions 1–10? Yes _____ No _____
    If yes, in what part of your body was the pain? _____

    B) If yes, was that symptom due to a physical illness or an accident? Yes _____ No _____

    C) Have you seen a doctor for that symptom? Yes _____ No _____

    D) If yes, what was the doctor's diagnosis? _____

12. A) Have you ever had a lot of trouble with excessive vomiting, at times other than during pregnancy? Yes _____ No _____

    B) If yes, was that symptom due to a physical illness or an accident? Yes _____ No _____

    C) Have you seen a doctor for that symptom? Yes _____ No _____

    D) If yes, what was the doctor's diagnosis? _____

13. A) During any pregnancy, did you vomit all through the pregnancy? Yes _____ No _____

    B) If yes, was that symptom due to a physical illness or an accident? Yes _____ No _____

    C) Have you seen a doctor for that symptom? Yes _____ No _____

    D) If yes, what was the doctor's diagnosis? _____

14. A) Have you ever had a lot of trouble with nausea (feeling sick to your stomach but not actually vomiting)? Yes _____ No _____

    B) If yes, was that symptom due to a physical illness or an accident? Yes _____ No _____

    C) Have you seen a doctor for that symptom? Yes _____ No _____

    D) If yes, what was the doctor's diagnosis? _____

15. A) Have you ever had a lot of trouble with loose bowels or diarrhea? Yes _____ No _____

    B) If yes, was that symptom due to a physical illness or an accident? Yes _____ No _____

    C) Have you seen a doctor for that symptom? Yes _____ No _____

    D) If yes, what was the doctor's diagnosis? _____

16. A) Have you ever had a lot of trouble with excessive gas or bloating of your stomach or abdomen? Yes _____ No _____

    B) If yes, was that symptom due to a physical illness or an accident? Yes _____ No _____

    C) Have you seen a doctor for that symptom? Yes _____ No _____

    D) If yes, what was the doctor's diagnosis? _____

(continued)

17. A) Have you found there were several kinds of foods that you couldn't eat because they made you ill? Yes _____ No _____
    B) If yes, was that symptom due to a physical illness or an accident? Yes _____ No _____
    C) Have you seen a doctor for that symptom? Yes _____ No _____
    D) If yes, what was the doctor's diagnosis? _____

18. A) Have you ever lost your vision in one or both eyes to the extent that you couldn't see anything at all for a few seconds or more? Yes _____ No _____
    B) If yes, was that symptom due to a physical illness or an accident? Yes _____ No _____
    C) Have you seen a doctor for that symptom? Yes _____ No _____
    D) If yes, what was the doctor's diagnosis? _____

19. A) Has your vision ever become blurred for some period (not including times when you needed glasses or a change in your glasses)? Yes _____ No _____
    B) If yes, was that symptom due to a physical illness or an accident? Yes _____ No _____
    C) Have you seen a doctor for that symptom? Yes _____ No _____
    D) If yes, what was the doctor's diagnosis? _____

20. A) Have you ever completely lost your hearing for a period of time? Yes _____ No _____
    B) If yes, was that symptom due to a physical illness or an accident? Yes _____ No _____
    C) Have you seen a doctor for that symptom? Yes _____ No _____
    D) If yes, what was the doctor's diagnosis? _____

21. A) Have you ever had trouble walking? Yes _____ No _____
    B) If yes, was that symptom due to a physical illness or an accident? Yes _____ No _____
    C) Have you seen a doctor for that symptom? Yes _____ No _____
    D) If yes, what was the doctor's diagnosis? _____

22. A) Have you ever lost feeling in an arm or a leg (at times other than when it had just fallen asleep or become numb from being in one position too long)? Yes _____ No _____
    B) If yes, was that symptom due to a physical illness or an accident? Yes _____ No _____
    C) Have you seen a doctor for that symptom? Yes _____ No _____
    D) If yes, what was the doctor's diagnosis? _____

(continued)

23. A) Have you ever been completely unable to move a part of your body for at least a few minutes? Yes _____ No _____
    B) If yes, was that symptom due to a physical illness or an accident? Yes _____ No _____
    C) Have you seen a doctor for that symptom? Yes _____ No _____
    D) If yes, what was the doctor's diagnosis? _____

24. A) Have you ever lost your voice for 30 minutes or more so that you couldn't speak above a whisper? Yes _____ No _____
    B) If yes, was that symptom due to a physical illness or an accident? Yes _____ No _____
    C) Have you seen a doctor for that symptom? Yes _____ No _____
    D) If yes, what was the doctor's diagnosis? _____

25. A) During the time since your 12th birthday, have you ever had a seizure or convulsion that caused you to become unconscious or caused your body to jerk uncontrollably? Yes _____ No _____
    B) If yes, was that symptom due to a physical illness or an accident? Yes _____ No _____
    C) Have you seen a doctor for that symptom? Yes _____ No _____
    D) If yes, what was the doctor's diagnosis? _____

26. A) Have you ever had fainting (or falling out) spells where you felt weak or dizzy and then passed out? Yes _____ No _____
    B) If yes, was that symptom due to a physical illness or an accident? Yes _____ No _____
    C) Have you seen a doctor for that symptom? Yes _____ No _____
    D) If yes, what was the doctor's diagnosis? _____

27. A) Have you ever been unconscious for any other reason? Yes _____ No _____
    B) If yes, was that symptom due to a physical illness or an accident? Yes _____ No _____
    C) Have you seen a doctor for that symptom? Yes _____ No _____
    D) If yes, what was the doctor's diagnosis? _____

28. A) Have you ever had a period of amnesia—that is, a period of several hours or days when you couldn't remember anything afterward about what had happened during that time? Yes _____ No _____
    B) If yes, was that symptom due to a physical illness or an accident? Yes _____ No _____
    C) Have you seen a doctor for that symptom? Yes _____ No _____
    D) If yes, what was the doctor's diagnosis? _____

(continued)

29. A) Have you ever had problems with double vision? Yes _____ No _____
    B) If yes, was that symptom due to a physical illness or an accident? Yes _____ No _____
    C) Have you seen a doctor for that symptom? Yes _____ No _____
    D) If yes, what was the doctor's diagnosis? _____

30. A) Have you ever had shortness of breath when you had not been exercising or exerting yourself? Yes _____ No _____
    B) If yes, was that symptom due to a physical illness or an accident? Yes _____ No _____
    C) Have you seen a doctor for that symptom? Yes _____ No _____
    D) If yes, what was the doctor's diagnosis? _____

31. A) Has your heart ever beat so hard that you could feel it pound in your chest? Yes _____ No _____
    B) If yes, was that symptom due to a physical illness or an accident? Yes _____ No _____
    C) Have you seen a doctor for that symptom? Yes _____ No _____
    D) If yes, what was the doctor's diagnosis? _____

32. A) Have you ever been bothered by dizziness? Yes _____ No _____
    B) If yes, was that symptom due to a physical illness or an accident? Yes _____ No _____
    C) Have you seen a doctor for that symptom? Yes _____ No _____
    D) If yes, what was the doctor's diagnosis? _____

33. A) Have you ever been bothered by periods of weakness—that is, when you could not lift or move things you could normally lift or move? Yes _____ No _____
    B) If yes, was that symptom due to a physical illness or an accident? Yes _____ No _____
    C) Have you seen a doctor for that symptom? Yes _____ No _____
    D) If yes, what was the doctor's diagnosis? _____

34. A) Have you ever been bothered a lot by blotchiness or discoloration of the skin? Yes _____ No _____
    B) If yes, was that symptom due to a physical illness or an accident? Yes _____ No _____
    C) Have you seen a doctor for that symptom? Yes _____ No _____
    D) If yes, what was the doctor's diagnosis? _____

35. A) Did you ever have a lot of trouble with a bad taste in your mouth or an excessively coated tongue? Yes _____ No _____
    B) If yes, was that symptom due to a physical illness or an accident? Yes _____ No _____

(continued)

184

C) Have you seen a doctor for that symptom? Yes _____ No _____
D) If yes, what was the doctor's diagnosis? _____

36. A) Did having to urinate too frequently ever cause you a lot of trouble? Yes _____ No _____
    B) If yes, was that symptom due to a physical illness or an accident? Yes _____ No _____
    C) Have you seen a doctor for that symptom? Yes _____ No _____
    D) If yes, what was the doctor's diagnosis? _____

37. A) Have you ever been bothered a lot by unpleasant numbness or tingling sensations? Yes _____ No _____
    B) If yes, was that symptom due to a physical illness or an accident? Yes _____ No _____
    C) Have you seen a doctor for that symptom? Yes _____ No _____
    D) If yes, what was the doctor's diagnosis? _____

38. A) Have you ever felt as though there were a lump in your throat that made it difficult to swallow? Yes _____ No _____
    B) If yes, was that symptom due to a physical illness or an accident? Yes _____ No _____
    C) Have you seen a doctor for that symptom? Yes _____ No _____
    D) If yes, what was the doctor's diagnosis? _____

39. A) Other than during your first year of menstruation, have your menstrual periods ever been irregular? Yes _____ No _____
    B) If yes, was that symptom due to a physical illness or an accident? Yes _____ No _____
    C) Have you seen a doctor for that symptom? Yes _____ No _____
    D) If yes, what was the doctor's diagnosis? _____

40. A) Have you ever had excessive bleeding with your menstrual periods? Yes _____ No _____
    B) If yes, was that symptom due to a physical illness or an accident? Yes _____ No _____
    C) Have you seen a doctor for that symptom? Yes _____ No _____
    D) If yes, what was the doctor's diagnosis? _____

How old were you when you were first bothered by symptoms described in items 1–40? Age first bothered _____

How old were you when you were last bothered by symptoms such as those described in Items 1–40? Age when last bothered _____

SCORING KEY FOR SOMATIC SYMPTOM QUESTIONNAIRE

Each item (1–40) is scored 0 or 1.

An item receives a score of 1 if <u>all</u> of the following are true:
1. Both statements A and C are checked <u>"yes."</u>
2. Statement B is checked <u>"no."</u>
3. Response to statement D suggests the symptom was medically unexplained (e.g., no or unknown diagnosis, tension, stress, nerves, etc.).

An item receives a score of 0 if any one of the above requirements is not true.

The total score is the sum of items 1–40.

Scores ≥ 6 suggest at least moderate somatization.

Instructions for Abbreviated Progressive Muscle Relaxation

The exercise involves tensing and releasing tension from a number of different muscle groups. Before we begin, I want to show you exactly what we'll be doing and give you a word of advice. When you tense each muscle group, be careful not to tense any muscle so tightly that it hurts. The goal of tensing is to help you focus your attention on each specific muscle group. You may only need to tighten the muscles slightly. Just tense them enough to feel the tension. Usually, tensing a muscle group slightly for about 5–8 seconds is sufficient to experience sensations of tension in that muscle group. The releasing of tension from each muscle group will last longer, about 60 seconds for each. Okay? The specific muscle groups to be tensed and released are:

1. *The forearms* (Therapist demonstrates tensing forearms and asks patient to follow)
2. *The upper arms or biceps* (Therapist and patient tense biceps)
3. *The lower legs* (Therapist and patient tense lower legs)
4. *The upper legs and buttocks* (Therapist and patient tense quadriceps and buttocks)
5. *The stomach* (Therapist and patient tense stomach)
6. *The chest and upper back* (Therapist and patient tense chest and upper back)
7. *The shoulders* (Therapist and patient raise shoulders)
8. *The neck* (Therapist and patient tense neck)

9. *The mouth and jaw* (Therapist and patient tense mouth and jaw)
10. *The eyes* (Therapist and patient shut eyes tightly)
11. *The lower forehead* (Therapist and patient tense lower forehead)
12. *The upper forehead* (Therapist and patient tense upper forehead)

[Next, the therapist tells the patient that the exercise will take about 20–30 minutes. The therapist reads the following script VERBATIM, while tensing and releasing his or her muscle groups along with the patient. No more than 8 seconds should be spent applying tension to any single muscle group.]

Find a comfortable position in the relaxation chair. We want all parts of your body to be completely supported by the chair so you can let your muscles relax completely and allow your body to sink into the chair.

(1) Create some tension in your lower arms by making fists with your hands and bending the fists inward toward the inside of your forearms. Notice the tension in your lower arms and hands. Now let your hands and lower arms go limp as you let go of the tension in them. Notice the sensations in your forearms and hands as the tension subsides and the muscles relax. Feel the difference between the tension of a moment ago and the relaxation in your forearms and hands now.

(2) Now create some tension in your upper arms by pulling your lower arms up, bending your elbow like you're doing a bicep curl. Notice the tension in your upper arms. Try to avoid tensing muscles in other parts of your body while you do this. Now relax your arms and let them drop down beside you. Notice the release of tension in your upper arms and feel the difference in comparison to the tension in them of a moment ago. Your arms may feel heavy, warm, and relaxed.

(3) Now create some tension in your lower legs by flexing your feet and pulling your toes towards your shins. Notice the tension in your feet, shins, and calf muscles. Now let go of the tension. Let your feet and legs relax. Feel the difference in the muscles as they relax from their tension of a moment ago.

(4) Now create some tension in your upper legs and rear end by pushing your feet against the floor, as though you were attempting to stand up, and tensing your buttocks. Notice the tension in your upper legs and buttocks. Now release the tension, and let your legs rest heavily on the chair. Let go of the tension. Notice the feeling of relaxation in your legs and buttocks.

(5) Now create some tension in your stomach by pulling your stomach in while at the same time trying to push it out. Now let the stomach go. Release the tension and breathe abdominally. Feel the sense of warmth across your stomach.

(6) Now create some tension around your chest and upper back by pulling your shoulder blades back as though you were trying to touch them together. Feel the tension across your chest and back. Now let the tension go. Notice the difference as the muscles in your chest and upper back relax.

(7) Now pull your shoulders up toward your ears. Experience the tension in your neck and shoulders. Now let the shoulders relax and drop down. Notice the difference as the tension subsides.

(8) Now create some tension around your neck by pulling your chin down toward the top of your chest while you also push the back of your neck into the headrest of the chair. Notice the tension around the back of your neck and head. Now let go of that tension and let your head lie back against the chair. Notice the sensations in your neck and the difference between tension and the absence of tension.

(9) Now create some tension around your mouth, jaw, and throat by clenching your teeth and pulling back the corners of your mouth back as though you were forcing a smile. Notice the tension. Now release the tension around your mouth, throat, and jaw. Experience the difference in feeling as you release the tension.

(10) Now create some tension around your eyes by squeezing your eyelids shut. Now release the tension from around your eyes. Notice the difference in sensations around your eyes during the tension and after the release of tension.

(11) Now create some tension in your lower forehead by frowning, bringing your eyebrows closer together. Feel the sensations of tension. Now release the tension. Let your eyebrows relax and notice the sensations you experience in your lower forehead as the tension subsides.

(12) Now create some tension across your upper forehead by raising your eyebrows and wrinkling your forehead. Now relax that area. Make the wrinkles on your forehead disappear. Let go of the tension in your forehead.

Now let your breathing become slow and regular. Let yourself experience the sensations that come when your muscles are relatively free from tension (30-second pause). Now take a moment and review each area of your body. If you notice any muscle tension in any area, tense that area ever so slightly and then release the tension. Let the muscles relax, loosen, and go limp. Just let your body sink down into the chair and relax.

Examining Thoughts

1. What is the evidence that supports this thought? (What makes me think it's true?)

2. What is the evidence against this thought?

3. Considering #1 and #2, is there another way of construing my original thought?

4. What would a caring and perceptive friend say to me about this thought?

5. What would I say to someone I care about who had this thought?

6. What is the effect of my believing in the truth and importance of the thought?

7. What could be the effect of changing my thinking?

8. What is the *worst* possible outcome connected with this thought? What would be the consequences for me?

9. What is the best possible outcome connected with this thought?

10. What is the most realistic outcome?

References

Aaron, L. A., Bradley, L. A., Alarcon, G. S., Triana-Alexander, M., Alexander R. W., Martin, M. Y., et al. (1997). Perceived physical and emotional trauma as precipitating events in fibromyalgia: Associations with health care seeking and disability status but not pain severity. *Arthritis and Rheumatism, 40,* 453–460.

Affleck, G., Urrows, S., Tennen, H., & Higgins, P. (1996). Sequential daily relations of sleep, pain intensity, and attention to pain among women with fibromyalgia. *Pain, 68,* 363–368.

Alexander, F. (1950). *Psychosomatic medicine.* New York: Norton.

Alfven, G., de la Torre, B., & Uvnas-Moberg, K. (1994). Depressed concentrations of oxytocin and cortisol in children with recurrent abdominal pain of non-organic pain. *Acta Paediatrica, 83,* 1076–1080.

Allen, L. A., Escobar, J. I., Lehrer, P. M., Gara, M. A., & Woolfolk, R. L. (2002). Psychosocial treatments for multiple unexplained physical symptoms: A review of the literature. *Psychosomatic Medicine, 64,* 939–950.

Allen, L. A., Gara, M. A., Escobar, J. I., Waitzkin, H., & Cohen-Silver, R. (2001). Somatization: A debilitating syndrome in primary care. *Psychosomatics, 42,* 63–67.

Allen, L. A., Woolfolk, R. L., Escobar, J. I., Gara, M. A., & Hamer, R. M. (2006). Cognitive-behavioral therapy for somatization disorder: A randomized controlled trial. *Archives of Internal Medicine, 166,* 1512–1518.

Allen, L. A., Woolfolk, R. L., & Gara, M. A. (2001). Cognitive behavior therapy for somatization disorder. *Psychosomatic Medicine, 63,* 93–94.

Allen, L. A., Woolfolk, R. L., Lehrer, P. M., Gara, M. A., & Escobar, J. I. (2001). Cognitive behavior therapy for somatization: A pilot study. *Journal of Behavior Therapy and Experimental Psychiatry, 32,* 53–62.

American Psychiatric Association. (1980). *Diagnostic and statistical manual of mental disorders* (3rd ed.). Washington, DC: Author.

191

American Psychiatric Association. (1987). *Diagnostic and statistical manual of mental disorders* (3rd ed., rev.). Washington, DC: Author.

American Psychiatric Association. (1994). *Diagnostic and statistical manual of mental disorders* (4th ed.). Washington, DC: Author.

Anderson, K. O., Dalton, C. B., Bradley, L. A., & Richter, J. E. (1989). Stress induces alteration of esophageal pressures in healthy volunteers and non-cardiac chest pain patients. *Digestive Diseases and Sciences, 34,* 83–91.

Apley, J., & Naish, N. (1958). Recurrent abdominal pains: A field study of 1,000 schoolchildren. *Archives of Disease in Childhood, 33,* 165–170.

Arnold, L. M., Keck, P. E., & Welge, J. A. (2000). Antidepressant treatment of fibromyalgia: A meta-analysis and review. *Psychosomatics, 41,* 104–113.

Arnold, L. M., Lu, Y., Crofford, L. J., Wohlreich, M., Detke, M. J., Iyengar, S., et al. (2004). A double-blind, multicenter trial comparing duloxetine with placebo in the treatment of fibromyalgia patients with or without major depressive disorder. *Arthritis and Rheumatism, 50,* 2974–2984.

Arnold, L. M., Rosen, A., Pritchett, Y. L., D'Souza, D. N., Goldstein, D. J., Iyengar, S., et al. (2005). A randomized, double-blind, placebo-controlled trial of duloxetine in the treatment of women with fibromyalgia with or without major depressive disorder. *Pain, 119,* 5–15.

Arnold, M. B. (1960). *Emotion and personality.* New York: Columbia University Press.

Arroyo, J. F., & Cohen, M. L. (1993). Abnormal responses to electrocutaneous stimulation in fibromyalgia. *Journal of Rheumatology, 20,* 1925–1931.

Avila, L. A., & Winston, M. (2003). Georg Groddeck: Originality and exclusion. *History of Psychiatry, 14,* 83–101.

Bagby, R. M., Parker, J. D., & Taylor, G. J. (1994). The twenty-item Toronto Alexithymia Scale—I. Item selection and cross-validation of the factor structure. *Journal of Psychosomatic Research, 38,* 23–32.

Bagby, R. M., Taylor, G. J., & Parker, J. D. (1994). The twenty-item Toronto Alexithymia Scale—II. Convergent, discriminant, and concurrent validity. *Journal of Psychosomatic Research, 38,* 33–40.

Bandura, A. (1986). *Social foundations of thought and action: A social cognitive theory.* Englewood Cliffs, NJ: Prentice-Hall.

Bargh, J. A., & Chartrand T. L. (1999). The unbearable automaticity of being. *American Psychologist, 54,* 462–479.

Barlow, D. H., & Craske, M. G. (1994). *Mastery of your anxiety and panic, II.* San Antonio, TX: Graywind/Psychological Corp.

Barsky, A. J. (1992). Amplification, somatization, and the somatoform disorders. *Psychosomatics, 33,* 28–34.

Barsky, A. J., & Ahern, D. K. (2004). Cognitive behavior therapy for hypochondriasis: A randomized controlled trial. *Journal of the American Medical Association, 291,* 1464–1470.

Barsky, A. J., & Borus, J. F. (1995). Somatization and medicalization in the era of managed care. *Journal of the American Medical Association, 274,* 1931–1934.

Barsky, A. J., & Borus, J. F. (1999). Functional somatic syndromes. *Annals of Internal Medicine, 130,* 910–921.

Barsky, A. J., Coeytaux, R. R., Sarnie, M. K., & Cleary, P. D. (1993). Hypochondriacal patients' beliefs about good health. *American Journal of Psychiatry,* *150,* 1085–1089.

Barsky, A. J., & Klerman, G. L. (1983). Overview: Hypochondriasis, bodily complaints, and somatic styles. *American Journal of Psychiatry, 140,* 273–283.

Barsky, A. J., Orav, E. J., & Bates, D. W. (2005). Somatization increases medical utilization and costs independent of psychiatric and medical comorbidity. *Archives of General Psychiatry, 62,* 903–910.

Barsky, A. J., Wyshak, G., & Klerman, G. L. (1990). The somatosensory amplification scale and its relationship to hypochondriasis. *Journal of Psychiatric Research, 24,* 323–334.

Barsky, A. J., Wyshak, G., & Klerman, G. L. (1992). Psychiatric comorbidity in DSM-III-R hypochondriasis. *Archives of General Psychiatry, 49,* 101–108.

Bass, C., & Murphy, M. (1991) Somatisation disorder in a British teaching hospital. *British Journal of Clinical Practice, 45,* 237–244

Baum, A., & Posluszny, D. M. (1999). Health psychology: Mapping biobehavioral contributions to health and illness. *Annual Review of Psychology, 50,* 137–163.

Beach, S. R. H., Fincham, F. D., & Katz, J. (1998). Marital therapy in the treatment of depression: Toward a third generation of therapy and research. *Clinical Psychology Review, 18,* 635–661.

Beck, A. T. (1976). *Cognitive therapy and the emotional disorders.* New York: International Universities Press.

Beck, A. T., Epstein, N., Brown, G., & Steer, R. A. (1988). An inventory for measuring clinical anxiety: Psychometric properties. *Journal of Consulting and Clinical Psychology, 56,* 893–897.

Beck, A. T., Rush, A. J., Shaw, B. F., & Emery, G. (1979). *Cognitive therapy of depression.* New York: Guilford Press.

Beck, A. T., Ward, C. H., Mendelson, M., Mock, J., & Erbaugh, J. (1961). An inventory for measuring depression. *Archives of General Psychiatry, 4,* 561–571.

Bennett, P., & Wilkinson, S. (1985). A comparison of psychological and medical treatment of the irritable bowel syndrome. *British Journal of Clinical Psychology, 24,* 215–216.

Berenbaum, H., Raghavan, C., Le, H.-N., Vernon, L. L., & Gomez, J. J. (2003). A taxonomy of emotional disturbances. *Clinical Psychology: Science and Practice, 10,* 206–226.

Bergner, M., Bobbitt, R. A., Carter, W. B., & Gilson, B. S. (1981). The Sickness Impact Profile: Development and final revision of a health status measure. *Medical Care, 19,* 787–805.

Bernstein, D. A., & Carlson, C. R. (1993). Progressive relaxation: Abbreviated methods. In P. M. Lehrer & R. L. Woolfolk (Eds.), *Principles and practice of stress management* (2nd ed., pp. 53–87). New York: Guilford Press.

Biddle, B. J. (1986). Recent developments in role theory. *Annual Review of Sociology, 12,* 67–92.

Black, D. R., Gleser, L. J., & Kooyers, K. J. (1990). A meta-analytic evaluation of couples weight-loss programs. *Health Psychology, 9,* 330–347.

Blakely, A. A., Howard, R. C., Sosich, R. M., Murdoch, J. C., Menkes, D. B., & Spears, G. F. S. (1991). Psychiatric symptoms, personality, and ways of coping in chronic fatigue syndrome. *Psychological Medicine, 21,* 347–362.

Blanchard, E. B., Greene, B., Scharff, L., & Schwarz-McMorris, S. P. (1993). Relaxation training as a treatment for irritable bowel syndrome. *Biofeedback and Self-Regulation, 18,* 125–132.

Blanchard, E. B., Schwarz, S. P., Suls, J. M., Gerardi, M. A., Scharff, L., Greene, B., et al. (1992). Two controlled evaluations of multi-component psychological treatment of irritable bowel syndrome. *Behaviour Research and Therapy, 30,* 175–189.

Bloch, S., & Reddaway, P. (1977). *Psychiatric terror.* New York: Basic Books.

Bombardier, C. H., & Buchwald, D. (1996). Chronic fatigue, chronic fatigue syndrome, and fibromyalgia: Disability and health-care use. *Medical Care, 34,* 924–930.

Bootzin, R. R, & Rider, S. P. (1997). Behavioral techniques and biofeedback for insomnia. In M. R. Pressman & W. C. Orr (Eds.), *Understanding sleep: The evaluation and treatment of sleep disorders* (pp. 315–338). Washington, DC: American Psychological Association.

Borkovec, T. D., & Costello, E. (1993). Efficacy of applied relaxation and cognitive-behavioral therapy in the treatment of generalized anxiety disorder. *Journal of Consulting and Clinical Psychology, 61,* 611–619.

Boss, J. M. N. (1979). The seventeenth-century transformation of the hysteric affection, and Sydenham's Baconian medicine. *Psychological Medicine, 9,* 221–234.

Boyce, P. M., Talley, N. J., Balaam, B., Koloski, N. A., & Truman, G. (2003). A randomized controlled trial of cognitive behavioral therapy, relaxation training, and routine clinical care for the irritable bowel syndrome. *American Journal of Gastroenterology, 98,* 2209–2218.

Breuer, J., & Freud, S. (1974). *Studies on hysteria* (J. Strachey & A. Strachey, Trans.). Harmondsworth, UK: Penguin. (Original work published 1895)

Briquet, P. (1859). *Traité clinique et thérapeutique de l'hystérie.* Paris: Bailliére & Fils.

Brown, F. W., Golding, J. M., & Smith, R., Jr. (1990). Psychiatric comorbidity in primary care somatization disorder. *Psychosomatic Medicine, 52,* 445–451.

Brown, R. J., Schrag, A., & Trimble, M. R. (2005). Dissociation, childhood interpersonal trauma, and family functioning in patients with somatization disorder. *American Journal of Psychiatry, 162,* 899–905.

Bucholz, K. K., Dinwiddie, S. H., Reich, T., Shayka, J. J., & Cloninger, C. R. (1993). Comparison of screening proposals for somatization disorder empirical analyses. *Comprehensive Psychiatry, 34,* 59–64.

Buchwald, D., & Garrity, D. (1994). Comparison of patients with chronic fatigue syndrome, fibromyalgia, and multiple chemical sensitivities. *Archives of Internal Medicine, 154,* 2049–2053.

Burckhardt, C. S., & Bjelle, A. (1996). Perceived control: A comparison of women with fibromyalgia, rheumatoid arthritis, and systemic lupus erythematosus using a Swedish version of the Rheumatology Attitudes Index. *Scandanavian Journal of Rheumatology, 25,* 300–306.

Bushbaum, M. (1975). Averaged evoked response augmenting/reducing in schizophrenia and affective disorders. *Association for Research in Nervous Mental Disease, 54,* 29–42.

Camilleri, M., & Choi, M. G. (1997). Irritable bowel syndrome. *Alimentary Pharmacological Therapy, 11,* 3–15.

Campo, J. V., & Fritsch, S. L. (1994). Somatization in children and adolescents. *Journal of the American Academy of Child and Adolescent Psychiatry, 33,* 1223–1235.

Campo, J. V., Jansen-McWilliams, L., Comer, D. M., & Kelleher, K. J. (1999). Somatization in pediatric primary care: Association with psychopathology, functional impairment, and use of services. *Journal of the American Academy of Child and Adolescent Psychiatry, 38,* 1093–1101.

Carette, J., Bell, M. J., Reynolds, W. J., Haraoui, B., McCain, G. A., Bykerk, V. P., et al. (1994). Comparison of amitriptyline, cyclobenzaprine, and placebo in the treatment of fibromyalgia: A randomized, double-blind clinical trial. *Arthritis and Rheumatism, 37,* 32–40.

Cartwright, S. A. (1981). Report on the diseases and physical peculiarities of the Negro race. In A. L. Caplan, H. T. Engelhardt, Jr., & J. J. McCartney (Eds.), *Concepts of health and disease: Interdisciplinary perspectives* (pp. 305–326). Reading, MA: Addison-Wesley. (Original work published 1851)

Chaturvedi, S. K., Maguire P., & Somashekar, B. S. (2006). Somatization in cancer. *International Review of Psychiatry, 18,* 49–54.

Chinese Medical Association & Nanjing Medical University. (1995). *Chinese classification of mental disorders* (2nd ed., rev.). Nanjing: Dong Nan University Press (in Chinese).

Clark, D. M., Salkovskis, P. M., Hackmann, A., Wells, A., Fennell, M., Ludgate, J., et al. (1998). Two psychological treatments for hypochondriasis. A randomised controlled trial. *British Journal of Psychiatry, 173,* 218–225.

Clark, M. R., Katon, W., Russo, J., Kith, P., Sintay, M., & Buchwald, D. (1995). Risk factors for symptom persistence in a 2½ year follow-up study. *American Journal of Medicine, 98,* 187–195.

Clark, S., Tindall, E., & Bennett, R. M. (1985). A double blind crossover trial of prednisone versus placebo in the treatment of fibrosis. *Journal of Rheumatology, 12,* 980–983.

Clauw, D. J. (1995). The pathogenesis of chronic pain and fatigue syndromes, with special reference to fibromyalgia. *Medical Hypotheses, 44,* 369–378.

Cleare, A. J., Heap, E., Malhi, G. S., Wessely, S., O'Keane, V., & Miell, J. (1999). Low-dose hydrocortisone in chronic fatigue syndrome: A randomized crossover trial. *Lancet, 353,* 455–458.

Cohen, S., & Herbert, T. B. (1996). Health psychology: Psychological factors and physical disease from the perspective of human psychoneuroimmunology. *Annual Review of Psychology, 47,* 113–142.

Corney, R. H., Stanton, R., Newell, R., Clare, A., & Fairclough, P. (1991). Behavioural psychotherapy in the treatment of irritable bowel syndrome. *Journal of Psychosomatic Research, 35,* 461–469.

Corruble, E., & Guelfi, J. D. (2000). Pain complaints in depressed inpatients. *Psychopathology, 33,* 307–309.

Coryell, W., & Norten, S. G. (1981). Briquet's syndrome (somatization disorder) and primary depression: Comparison of background and outcome. *Comprehensive Psychiatry, 22,* 249–256.

Craig, T. K. J., Cox, A. D., & Klein, K. (2002). Intergenerational transmission of somatization behaviour: A study of chronic somatizers and their children. *Psychological Medicine, 32,* 805–816.

Creed, F., & Barsky, A. (2004). A systematic review of the epidemiology of somatisation disorder and hypochondriasis. *Journal of Psychosomatic Research, 56,* 391–408.

Creed, F., Fernandes, L., Guthrie, E., Palmer, S., Ratcliffe, J., Read, N., et al. (2003). The cost-effectiveness of psychotherapy and paroxetine for severe irritable bowel syndrome. *Gastroenterology, 124,* 303–317.

Crofford, L. J., Rowbotham, M. C., Mease, P. J., Russell, I. J., Dworkin, R. H., Corbin, A. E., et al. (2005). Pregabalin for the treatment of fibromyalgia syndrome: Results of a randomized, double-blind, placebo-controlled trial. *Arthritis and Rheumatism, 52,* 1264–1273.

Crowne, D. P., & Marlowe, D. (1960). A new scale of social desirability independent of psychopathology. *Journal of Consulting Psychology, 24,* 349–354.

Cyr, J. J., McKenna-Foley, J. M., & Peacock, E. (1985). Factor structure of the SCL-90–R: Is there one? *Journal of Personality Assessment, 49,* 571–578.

Danner, D. D., Snowdon, D. A., & Friesen, W. V. (2001). Positive emotions in early life and longevity: Findings from the nun study. *Journal of Personality and Social Psychology, 80,* 804–813.

Deale, A., Chalder, T., Marks, I., & Wessely, S. (1997). Cognitive behavior therapy for chronic fatigue syndrome: A randomized controlled trial. *American Journal of Psychiatry, 154,* 408–414.

Deale, A., Kaneez, A., Chalder, T., & Wessely S. (2001). Long-term outcome of cognitive behavior therapy versus relaxation therapy for chronic fatigue syndrome: A 5-year follow-up study. *American Journal of Psychiatry, 158,* 2038–2041.

Deary, I. J., Scott, S., & Wilson, J. A. (1997). Neuroticism, alexithymia and medically unexplained symptoms. *Personality and Individual Differences, 22,* 551–564.

de Bruin, A. F., Buys, M., de Witte, L. P., & Diederiks, J. P. (1994). The Sickness Impact Profile: SIP68, a short generic version. First evaluation of the reliability and reproducibility. *Journal of Clinical Epidemiology, 47,* 863–871.

de Bruin, A. F., Diederiks, J. P., de Witte, L. P., Stevens, F. C., & Philipsen, H. (1997). Assessing the responsiveness of a functional status measure: The Sickness Impact Profile versus the SIP68. *Journal of Clinical Epidemiology, 50,* 529–540.

De Gucht, V., & Heiser, W. (2003). Alexithymia and somatisation: Quantitative review of the literature. *Journal of Psychosomatic Research, 54,* 425–434.

DeLongis, A., Folkman, S., & Lazarus, R. S. (1988). The impact of daily stress on health and mood: Psychological and social resources as mediators. *Journal of Personality and Social Psychology 54,* 486–495.

Demitrack, M. A., Dale, J. K., Straus, S. E., Laue, L., Listwak, S. J., Kruesi, M. J., et al. (1991). Evidence for impaired activation of the hypothalamic-pituitary-adrenal axis in patients with chronic fatigue syndrome. *Journal of Clinical Endocrinology Metabolism, 73,* 1224–1234.

Derakshan, N., & Eysenck, M. W. (1999). Are repressors self-deceivers or other deceivers? *Cognition and Emotion, 13,* 1–17.

Derogatis, L. R. (1983). *SCL-90-R. Administration, scoring and procedures. Manual-II.* Towson, MD: Clinical Psychometric Research.

Deshields, T. L., Tait, R. C., Gfeller, J. D., & Chibnall, J. T. (1995). Relationship between social desirability and self-report in chronic pain patients. *Clinical Journal of Pain, 11,* 189–193.

Dickinson, W. P., Dickinson, L. M., deGruy, F. V., Main, D. S., Candib, L. M., & Rost, K. (2003). A randomized clinical trial of a care recommendation letter intervention for somatization in primary care. *Annals of Family Medicine, 1,* 228–235.

Dongier, M. (1983). Briquet and Briquet's syndrome viewed from France. *Canadian Journal of Psychiatry, 6,* 422–427.

Drewes, A. M., Andreasen, A., Jennum, P., & Nielson, K. D. (1991). Zopiclone in the treatment of sleep abnormalities in fibromyalgia. *Scandinavian Journal of Rheumatology, 20,* 288–293.

Drossman, D. A., Leserman, J., Nachman, G., Li, Z. M., Gluck, H., Toomey, T. C., et al. (1990). Sexual and physical abuse in women with functional or organic gastrointestinal disorders. *Annals of Internal Medicine, 113,* 828–833.

Drossman, D. A., Li, Z., Andruzzi, E., Temple, R. D., Talley, N. J., Thompson, W. G., et al. (1993). U.S. householder survey of functional gastrointestinal disorders: Prevalence, sociodemography and health impact. *Digestive Disease Science, 38,* 1569–1580.

Drossman, D. A., Toner, B. B., Whitehead, W. E., Diamant, N. E., Dalton, C. B., Duncan, S., et al. (2003). Cognitive-behavioral therapy versus education and desipramine versus placebo for moderate to severe functional bowel disorders. *Gastroenterology, 125,* 19–31.

Drossman, D. A., Whitehead, W. E., & Camilleri, M. (1997). Medical position statement: Irritable bowel syndrome. *Gastroenterology, 112,* 2118–2119.

Ehde, D. M., & Holm, J. E. (1992). Stress and headache: Comparisons of migraine, tension, and headache-free subjects. *Headache Quarterly, 3,* 54–60.

Ekman, P. (1992). An argument for basic emotions. *Cognition and Emotion, 6,* 169–200.

Ellis, A. (1962). *Reason and emotion in psychotherapy.* Secaucus, NJ: Citadel Press.

Elwan, O., Abdella, M., el Bayad, A. B., & Hamdy, S. (1991). Hormonal changes in headache patients. *Journal of Neurological Science, 106,* 75–81.

Engel, G. L. (1959). Psychogenic pain and the pain-prone patient. *American Journal of Medicine, 26,* 899–918.

Engel, G. L. (1977). The need for a new medical model: A challenge for biomedicine. *Science, 196,* 129–136.

Epstein, S. A., Kay, G., Clauw, D., Heaton, R., Klein, D., Krupp, L., et al. (1999). Psychiatric disorders in patients with fibromyalgia: A multicenter investigation. *Psychosomatics, 40,* 57–63.

Escobar, J. I., Burnam, M. A., Karno, M., Forsythe, A., & Golding J. M. (1987). Somatization in the community. *Archives of General Psychiatry, 44*, 713–718.

Escobar, J. I., Gara, M. A., Diaz-Martinez, A. M., Interian, A., Warman M., Allen, L. A., et al. (2006). *Effectiveness of a brief intervention for unexplained physical symptoms in primary care.* Manuscript submitted for publication.

Escobar, J. I., Gara, M., Waitzkin, H., Silver, R. C., Holman, A., & Compton, W. (1998). DSM-IV hypochondriasis in primary care. *General Hospital Psychiatry, 20*, 155–159.

Escobar, J. I., Golding, J. M., Hough, R. L., Karno, M., Burnam, M. A., & Wells, K. B. (1987). Somatization in the community: Relationship to disability and use of services. *American Journal of Public Health, 77*, 837–843.

Escobar, J. I., Rubio-Stipec, M., Canino, G., & Karno, M. (1989). Somatic Symptom Index (SSI): A new and abridged somatization construct. *Journal of Nervous and Mental Disease, 177*, 140–146.

Escobar, J. I., Waitzkin, H., Silver, R. C., Gara, M., & Holman, A. (1998). Abridged somatization: A study in primary care. *Psychosomatic Medicine, 60*, 466–472.

Evans, P. R., Bennett, E. J., Bak, Y. T., Tennent, C. C., & Kellow, J. E. (1996). Jejunal sensorimotor dysfunction in irritable bowel syndrome: Clinical and psychosocial features. *Gastroenterology, 110*, 393–404.

Evans, R. (1992). Some observations on whiplash injuries. *Neurologic Clinics, 10*, 975–997.

Fabrega, H. (1991). Somatization in cultural and historical perspective. In L. J. Kirmayer & J. M. Robbins (Eds.), *Current concepts of somatization* (pp. 181–199). Washington, DC: American Psychiatric Press.

Fabrega, H., Mezzich, J., Jacob, R., & Ulrich, R. (1988). Somatoform disorder in psychiatric setting: Systematic comparisons with depression and anxiety disorders. *Journal of Nervous and Mental Disease, 176*, 431–439.

Falconer, W. (1788). *A dissertation on the influence of the passions upon the disorders of the body.* London.

Fallon, B. A. (2004). Pharmacotherapy of somatoform disorders. *Journal of Psychosomatic Research, 56*, 455–460.

Feighner, J. P., Robins, E., Guze, S. B., Woodruff, R. A., Winokur, R., & Munoz, R. (1972). Diagnostic criteria for use in psychiatric research. *Archives of General Psychiatry, 26*, 57–63.

Ferraccioli, G., Ghirelli, L., Scita, F., Nolli, M., Mozzani, M., Fontana, S., et al. (1987). EMG-biofeedback training in fibromyalgia syndrome. *Journal of Rheumatology, 14*, 820–825.

Fink, P. (1992). Surgery and medical treatment in persistent somatizing patients. *Journal of Psychosomatic Research, 36*, 439–447.

Fink, P. (1995). Psychiatric illness in patients with persistent somatisation. *British Journal of Psychiatry, 166*, 93–99.

Fink, P., Sorensen, L., Engberg, M., Holm, M., & Munk-Jorgensen, P. (1999). Somatization in primary care: Prevalence, health care utilization, and general practitioner recognition. *Psychosomatics, 40*, 330–338.

First, M. B., Spitzer, R. L., Gibbon, M., & Williams, J. B. W. (1997). *Structured clinical interview for DSM-IV axis I disorders (SCID-I)*. Washington, DC: American Psychiatric Press.

Fishbain, D. A. (1994). Secondary gain concept. Definition problems and its abuse in medical practice. *American Pain Society Journal, 3*, 264–273.

Fishbain, D. A. (1998). Somatization, secondary gain, and chronic pain: Is there a relationship? *Current Pain and Headache Reports, 2*, 101–108.

Ford, M. J., Miller, P. M., Eastwood, J., & Eastwood, M. A. (1987). Life events, psychiatric illness and the irritable bowel syndrome. *Gut, 28*, 160–165.

Fordyce, W. E. (1976). *Behavioral methods for chronic pain and illness*. St. Louis, MO: Mosby.

Fors, E. A., Sexton, H., & Gotestam, K. G. (2002). The effect of guided imagery and amitriptyline on daily fibromyalgia pain: A prospective, randomized, controlled trial. *Journal of Psychiatric Research, 36*, 179–187.

Foucault, M. (1965). *Madness and civilization: A history of insanity in the age of reason* (R. Howard, Trans.). New York: Pantheon. (Original work published 1961)

Fredrickson, B. L., & Levenson, R. W. (1998). Positive emotions speed recovery from the cardiovascular sequelae of negative emotions. *Cognition and Emotion, 12*, 191–220.

Freedman, R. R., & Woodward, S. (1992). Behavioral treatment of menopausal hot flushes: Evaluation by ambulatory monitoring. *American Journal of Obstetrics and Gynecology, 167*, 436–439.

Frese, M. (1999). Social support as a moderator of the relationship between work stressors and psychological dysfunctioning: A longitudinal study with objective measures. *Journal of Occupational Health Psychology, 4*, 179–192.

Fried, R. (1993). The role of respiration in stress and stress control: Toward a theory of stress as a hypoxic phenomenon. In P. M. Lehrer & R. L. Woolfolk (Eds.), *Principles and practice of stress management* (2nd ed., pp. 301–331). New York: Guilford Press.

Fritz, G. K., Fritsch, S., & Hagino, O. (1997). Somatoform disorders in children and adolescents: A review of the past 10 years. *Child and Adolescent Psychiatry, 36*, 1329–1338.

Fukuda, K., Straus, S. E., Hickie, I., Sharpe, M. C., Dobbins, J. G., & Komaroff, A. (1994). The chronic fatigue syndrome: A comprehensive approach to its definition and study. *Annals of Internal Medicine, 121*, 953–959.

Fulcher, K. Y., & White, P. D. (1997). Randomised controlled trial of graded exercise in patients with the chronic fatigue syndrome. *British Medical Journal, 341*, 1647–1652.

Galovski, T. E., & Blanchard, E. B. (1998). The treatment of irritable bowel syndrome with hypnotherapy. *Applied Psychophysiology and Biofeedback, 23*, 219–232.

Gara, M. A., Rosenberg, S., & Woolfolk, R. L. (1993). Patient identity in major depression. *Depression, 1*, 257–262.

Garber, J., Walker, L. S., & Zeman, J. (1991). Somatization symptoms in a community sample of children and adolescents: Further validation of the Children's Somatization Inventory. *Psychological Assessment, 3*, 588–595.

Garber, J., Zeman, J., & Walker, L. S. (1990). Recurrent abdominal pain in children: Psychiatric diagnoses and parental psychopathology. *Journal of the American Academy of Child and Adolescent Psychiatry, 29,* 648–656.

Garcia-Campayo, J. J., Sanz-Carrillo, C., Perez-Echeverria, M. J., Campos, R., & Lobo, A. (1996). Screening of somatization disorder: Validation of the Spanish version of the Othmer and DeSouza test. *Acta Psychiatrica Scandinavica, 94,* 411–415.

Gardner, W. N., & Bass, C. (1989). Hyperventilation in clinical practice. *British Journal of Hospital Medicine, 41,* 73–81.

Gatchel, R. J. (2004). Psychosocial factors that can influence the self-assessment of function. *Journal of Occupational Rehabilitation, 14,* 197–206.

Gendlin, E. T. (1981). *Focusing* (2nd ed.). New York: Bantam Books.

Gendreau, R. M., Thorn, M. D., Gendreau, J. F., Kranzler, J. D., Ribeiro, S., Gracely, R. H., et al. (2005). Efficacy of milnacipran in patients with fibromyalgia. *Journal of Rheumatology, 32,* 1975–1985.

Gijswijt-Hofstra, M., & Porter, R. (Eds.). (2001). *Cultures of neurasthenia: From Beard to the First World War.* Amsterdam: Rodopi.

Goldenberg, D. L., Simms, R. W., Geiger, A., & Komaroff, A. K. (1990). High frequency of fibromyalgia in patients with chronic fatigue seen in a primary care practice. *Arthritis and Rheumatism, 33,* 381–387.

Golding, J. M., Smith, G. R., & Kashner, M. (1991). Does somatization disorder occur in men?: Clinical characteristics of women and men with multiple unexplained physical symptoms. *Archives of General Psychiatry, 48,* 231–235.

Greenberg, L. S. (2002). *Emotion-focused therapy: Coaching clients to work through their feelings.* Washington, DC: American Psychological Association.

Greenberg, L. S., & Watson, J. C. (2005). *Emotion-focused therapy for depression.* Washington, DC: American Psychological Association.

Greene, B., & Blanchard, E. D. (1994). Cognitive therapy for irritable bowel syndrome. *Journal of Consulting and Clinical Psychology, 62,* 576–582.

Greenwood, K. A, Thurston, R., Rumble, M., Waters, S. J., & Keefe, F. J. (2003). Anger and persistent pain: Current status and future directions. *Pain, 103,* 1–5.

Grob, G. N. (1991). *From asylum to community. Mental health policy in modern America.* Princeton, NJ: Princeton University Press.

Groddeck, G. (1977). *The meaning of illness.* London: Hogarth Press.

Gureje, O., & Simon, G. E. (1999). The natural history of somatization in primary care. *Psychological Medicine, 29,* 669–676.

Gureje, O., Simon, G. E., Ustun, T. B., & Goldberg, D. P. (1997). Somatization in cross-cultural perspective: A World Health Organization study in primary care. *American Journal of Psychiatry, 154,* 989–995.

Gureje, O., Ustun, T. B., & Simon, G. E. (1997). The syndrome of hypochondriasis: A cross-national study of primary care. *Psychological Medicine, 27,* 1001–1010.

Guthrie, E., Creed, F., Dawson, D., & Tomenson, B. (1991). A controlled trial of psychological treatment for the irritable bowel syndrome. *Gastroenterology, 100,* 450–457.

Guy, W. (1976). *ECDEU assessment manual for psychopharmacology*. Washington, DC: U.S. Department of Health, Education, and Welfare.

Guze, S. B. (1967). The diagnosis of hysteria: What are we trying to do? *American Journal of Psychiatry, 124*, 491–498.

Guze, S. B., & Perley, M. J. (1963). Observations on the natural history of hysteria. *American Journal of Psychiatry, 119*, 960–965.

Guze, S. B., Woodruff, R. A., & Clayton, P. J. (1972). Sex, age, and the diagnosis of hysteria (Briquet's syndrome). *American Journal of Psychiatry, 129*, 745–748.

Haanen, H. C., Hoenderdos, H. T., van Romunde, L. K., Hop, W. C., Mallee, C., Terwiel, J. P., et al. (1991). Controlled trial of hypnotherapy in the treatment of refractory fibromyalgia. *Journal of Rheumatology, 18*, 72–75.

Hacking, I. (1995). *Rewriting the soul: Multiple personality and the sciences of memory*. Princeton, NJ: Princeton University Press.

Hacking, I. (1999). *The social construction of what?* Cambridge, MA: Harvard University Press.

Hamaguchi, T., Kano, M., Rikimaru, H., Kanazawa, M., Itoh, M., Yanai, K., et al. (2004). Brain activity during distention of the descending colon in humans. *Neurogastroenterology and Motility, 16*, 299–309.

Hamilton, M. A. (1959). The assessment of anxiety states by rating. *British Journal of Medical Psychology, 32*, 50–55.

Hamilton, M. A. (1960). A rating scale for depression. *Journal of Neurology, Neurosurgery and Psychiatry, 23*, 56–62.

Hamilton, M. A. (1967). Development of a rating scale for primary depressive illness. *British Journal of Social and Clinical Psychology, 6*, 278–296.

Harber, V. J., & Sutton, J. R. (1984). Endorphins and exercise. *Sports Medicine, 1*, 154–171.

Hardt, J., Gerbershagen, H. U., & Franke, P. (2000). The symptom check-list, SCL-90–R: Its use and characteristics in chronic pain patients. *European Journal of Pain, 4*, 137–148.

Harrop-Griffiths, J., Katon, W., Walker, E., Holm, L., Russo, J., & Hickok, L. (1988). The association between chronic pelvic pain, psychiatric diagnoses, and childhood sexual abuse. *Obstetrics and Gynecology, 71*, 589–594.

Harvey, R. F., Salih, S. Y., & Read, A. E. (1983). Organic and functional disorders in 2000 gastroenterology outpatients. *Lancet, 1*, 632–634.

Hayes, S. C., Strosahl, K. D., & Wilson K. G. (1999). *Acceptance and commitment therapy: An experiential approach to behavior change*. New York: Guilford Press.

Heckman, T. G., Heckman, B. D., Kochman, A., Sikkema, K. J., Surh, J., & Goodkin, K. (2002). Psychological symptoms among persons 50 years of age and older living with HIV disease. *Aging and Mental Health, 6*, 121–128.

Heymann-Monnikes, I., Arnold, R., Florin, I., Herda, C., Melfsen, S., & Monnikes, H. (2000). The combination of medical treatment plus multicomponent behavioral therapy is superior to medical treatment alone in the therapy of irritable bowel syndrome. *American Journal of Gastroenterology, 95*, 981–994.

Hiller, W., Fichter, M. M., & Rief, W. (2003). A controlled treatment study of somatoform disorders including analysis of healthcare utilization and cost-effectiveness. *Journal of Psychosomatic Research, 54*, 369–380.

Hiller, W., Rief, W., & Fichter, M. M. (2002). Dimensional and categorical approaches to hypochondriasis. *Psychological Medicine, 32*, 707–718.

Hobbis, I. C., Turpin, G., & Read, N. W. (2002). A re-examination of the relationship between abuse experience and functional bowel disorders. *Gastroenterology, 37*, 423–430.

Holroyd, K. A. (2002). Assessment and psychological management of recurrent headache disorders. *Journal of Consulting and Clinical Psychology, 70*, 656–677.

Hotopf, M., Carr, S., Mayou, R., Wadsworth, M., & Wessely, S. (1998). Why do children have chronic abdominal pain, and what happens to them when they grow up?: Population based cohort study. *British Medical Journal, 316*, 1196–1200.

Hudson, J. I., Arnold, L. M., Keck, P. E., Achenbach, M. B., & Pope, H. G. (2004). Family study of affective spectrum disorder and fibromyalgia. *Biological Psychiatry, 56*, 884–891.

Izard, C. E. (1993). Four systems for emotion activation: Cognitive and noncognitive processes. *Psychological Review, 100*, 68–90.

Jackson, J. L., O'Malley, P. G., Tomkins, G., Balden, E., Santoro, J., & Kroenke, K. (2000). Treatment of functional gastrointestinal disorders with antidepressant medications: A meta-analysis. *American Journal of Medicine, 108*, 65–72.

Jacobson, E. (1938). *Progressive relaxation.* Chicago: University of Chicago Press.

Jailwala, J., Imperiale, T. F., & Kroenke, K. (2000). Pharmacologic treatment of the irritable bowel syndrome: A systematic review of randomized, controlled trials. *Annals of Internal Medicine, 133*, 136–147.

James, L., Gordon, E., Kraiuhin, C., Howson, A., & Meares, R. (1990). Augmentation of auditory evoked potentials in somatization disorder. *Journal of Psychosomatic Research, 24*, 155–163.

Jamner, L. D., Schwartz, G. E., & Leigh, H. (1988). The relationship between repressive and defensive coping styles and monocyte, eosinophile, and serum glucose levels: Support for the opiod peptide hypothesis of repression. *Psychosomatic Medicine, 50*, 567–575.

Jason, L. A., Richman, J. A., Rademaker, A. W., Jordan, K. M., Plioplys, A. V., Taylor, R. R., et al. (1999). A community-based study of chronic fatigue syndrome. *Archives of Internal Medicine, 159*, 2129–2137.

Johansson, F. (1982). Differences in serum cortisol concentrations in organic and psychogenic chronic pain syndromes. *Journal of Psychosomatic Research, 26*, 351–358.

Kashner, T. M., Rost, K., Cohen, B., Anderson, M., & Smith, G. R. (1995). Enhancing the health of somatization disorder patients: Effectiveness of short-term group therapy. *Psychosomatics, 36*, 462–470.

Katon, W., Lin, E., Von Korff, M., Russo, J., Lipscomb, P., & Bush, T. (1991). Somatization: A spectrum of severity. *American Journal of Psychiatry, 148*, 34–40.

Katon, W., Sullivan, M., & Walker E. (2001). Medical symptoms without identified pathology: Relationship to psychiatric disorders, childhood and adult trauma, and personality traits. *Annals of Internal Medicine, 134,* 917–925.

Katon, W. J., Von Korff, M., & Lin, E. (1992). Panic disorder: Relationship to high medical utilization. *American Journal of Medicine, 92,* 7S–11S.

Keefe, F. J., Caldwell, D. S., Baucom, D., Salley, A., Robinson, E., Timmons, K., et al. (1996). Spouse-assisted coping skills training in the management of osteoarthritic knee pain. *Arthritis Care and Research, 9,* 279–291.

Keel, P. J., Bodoky, C., Gerhard, U., & Muller, W. (1998). Comparison of integrated group therapy and group relaxation training for fibromyalgia. *Clinical Journal of Pain, 14,* 232–238.

Kelly, G. A. (1955). *The psychology of personal constructs.* New York: Norton.

Kennedy-Moore, E., & Watson, J. C. (1999). *Expressing emotion: Myths, realities, and therapeutic strategies.* New York: Guilford Press.

Kern, M. K., & Shaker, R. (2002). Cerebral cortical registration of subliminal visceral stimulation. *Gastroenterology, 122,* 290–298.

Kihlstrom, J. F., & Canter Kihlstrom, L. (1999). Self, sickness, somatization, and systems of care. In R. J. Contrada & R. D. Ashmore (Eds.), *Self, identity, and physical health: Interdisciplinary exploration* (pp. 23–42). New York: Oxford University Press.

King, A. C., Taylor, C. B., Albright, C. A., & Haskell, W. L. (1990). The relationship between repressive and defensive coping styles and blood pressure responses in healthy, middle-aged men and women. *Journal of Psychosomatic Research, 34,* 461–471.

King, D., Devine, D. P., Vierck, C. J., Rodgers, J., & Yezierski, R. P. (2003). Differential effects of stress on escape and reflex responses to nociceptive thermal stimuli in the rat. *Brain Research, 987,* 214–222.

King, S. J., Wessel, J., Bhambhani, Y., Sholter, D., & Maksymowych, W. (2002). The effects of exercise and education, individually or combined, in women with fibromyalgia. *Journal of Rheumatology, 29,* 2620–2627.

Kirmayer, L. J. (1984). Culture, affect and somatization, I. *Transcultural Psychiatric Research Review 21,* 159–188.

Kirmayer, L. J. (2001). Cultural variations in the clinical presentation of depression and anxiety: Implications for diagnosis and treatment. *Journal of Clinical Psychiatry, 62* (Suppl. 13), 22–28.

Kirmayer, L. J., & Robbins, J. M. (1991). Three forms of somatization in primary care: Prevalence, co-occurrence, and sociodemographic characteristics. *Journal of Nervous and Mental Disease, 179,* 647–655.

Kirmayer, L. J., & Robbins, J. M. (1996). Patients who somatize in primary care: A longitudinal study of cognitive and social characteristics. *Psychological Medicine, 26,* 937–951.

Kirmayer, L. J., Robbins, J. M., & Paris, J. (1994). Somatoform disorders: Personality and the social matrix of somatic distress. *Journal of Abnormal Psychology, 103,* 125–136.

Kirmayer, L. J., Young, A., & Robbins, J. M. (1994). Symptom attribution in cultural perspective. *Canadian Journal of Psychiatry, 39,* 584–595.

Klein, K. B. (1988). Controlled treatment trials in the irritable bowel syndrome: A critique. *Gastroenterology, 95,* 232–241.

Kleinman, A. (1982). Neurasthenia and depression: A study of somatization and culture in China. *Culture, Medicine, and Psychiatry, 6,* 117–190.

Kroenke, K., Arrington, M. E., & Mangelsdorff, A. D. (1990). The prevalence of symptoms in medical outpatients and the adequacy of therapy. *Archives of Internal Medicine, 150,* 1685–1689.

Kroenke, K., Messina, N., Benattia, I., Graepel, J., & Musgnung, J. (2006). Venlafaxine extended release in the short-term treatment of depressed and anxious primary care patients with multisomatoform disorder. *Journal of Clinical Psychiatry, 67,* 72–80.

Kroenke, K., Spitzer, R. L., deGruy, F. V., Hahn, S. R., Linzer, M., Williams, J. B., et al. (1997). Multisomatoform disorder: An alternative to undifferentiated somatoform disorder for the somatizing patient in primary care. *Archives of General Psychiatry, 54,* 352–358.

Kroenke, K., Spitzer, R. L., deGruy, F. V., & Swindle, R. (1998). A symptom checklist to screen for somatoform disorders in primary care. *Psychosomatics, 39,* 263–272.

Kroenke, K., Spitzer, R. L., & Williams, J. B. (2002). The PHQ-15: Validity of a new measure for evaluating the severity of somatic symptoms. *Psychosomatic Medicine, 64,* 258–266.

Kutchins, H., & Kirk, S. A. (1997). *Making us crazy: DSM: The psychiatric bible and the creation of mental disorders.* New York: Free Press.

Lackner, J. M., Gudleski, G. D., & Blanchard, E. B. (2004). Beyond abuse: The association among parenting style, abdominal pain, and somatization in IBS patients. *Behaviour Research and Therapy, 42,* 41–56.

Lane, R. D., Sechrest, L., Reidel, R., Shapiro, D. E., & Kaszniak, A. W. (2000). Pervasive emotion recognition deficit common to alexithymia and the repressive coping style. *Psychosomatic Medicine, 62,* 492–501.

Lautenbacher, S., Rollman, G. B., & McCain, G. A. (1994). Multi-method assessment of experimental and clinical pain in patients with fibromyalgia. *Pain, 59,* 418–421.

Lazarus, R. S. (1966). *Psychological stress and the coping process.* New York: McGraw-Hill.

Lazarus, R. S. (1994). *Emotion and adaptation.* New York: Oxford University Press.

LeDoux, J. E. (1995). Emotion: Clues from the brain. *Annual Review of Psychology, 46,* 209–235.

LeDoux, J. E. (1996). *The emotional brain: The mysterious underpinnings of emotional life.* New York: Simon & Schuster.

Lehrer, P. M. (1982). How to relax and how not to relax: A re-evaluation of the work of Edmund Jacobson. *Behaviour Research and Therapy, 20,* 417–428.

Lehrer, P. M., Sime, W. E., & Woolfolk, R. L. (Eds.). (in press). *Principles and practice of stress management* (3rd ed.). New York: Guilford Press.

Lehrer, P. M., & Woolfolk, R. L. (1993). Research on clinical issues in stress management. In P. M. Lehrer & R. L. Woolfolk (Eds.), *Principles and practice of stress management* (2nd ed., pp. 521–538). New York: Guilford Press.

Leong, S. A., Barghout, V., Birnbaum, H. G., Thibeault, C. E., Ben-Hamadi, R., Frech, F., et al. (2003). The economic consequences of irritable bowel syndrome: A U.S. employer perspective. *Archives of Internal Medicine, 163,* 929–935.

Lidbeck, J. (1997). Group therapy for somatization disorders in general practice: Effectiveness of a short cognitive-behavioural treatment model. *Acta Psychiatrica Scandinavica, 96,* 14–24.

Lidbeck, J. (2003). Group therapy for somatization disorders in primary care: Maintenance of treatment goals of short cognitive-behavioural treatment one-and-a-half-year follow-up. *Acta Psychiatrica Scandinavica, 107,* 449–456.

Lieb, R., Zimmermann, P., Friis, R. H., Mofler, M., Tholen, S., & Wittchen, H. U. (2002). The natural course of DSM-IV somatoform disorders and syndromes among adolescents and young adults: A prospective-longitudinal community study. *European Psychiatry, 17,* 321–331.

Liebman, W. M. (1978). Recurrent abdominal pain in children: A retrospective survey of 119 patients. *Clinical Pediatrics, 17,* 149–153.

Lin, E. H., Katon, W., Von Korff, M., Bush, T., Lipscomb, P., Russo, J., et al. (1991). Frustrating patients: Physician and patient perspectives among distressed high users of medical services. *Journal of General Internal Medicine, 6,* 241–246.

Lindeman, M., Saari, S., Verkasalo, M., & Prytz, H. (1996). Traumatic stress and its risk factors among peripheral victims of the M/S Estonia Disaster. *European Psychologist, 4,* 255–270.

Linehan, M. M. (1993). *Cognitive-behavioral treatment of borderline personality disorder.* New York: Guilford Press.

Linton, S. J. (1994). Chronic back pain: Integrating psychological and physical therapy—an overview. *Behavioral Medicine, 20,* 101–104.

Linton, S. J. (2000). A review of psychological risk factors in back and neck pain. *Spine, 25,* 1148–1156.

Lipowski, Z. J. (1988). Somatization: The concept and its clinical application. *American Journal of Psychiatry, 145,* 1358–1368.

Liu, G., Clark, M. R., & Eaton, W. W. (1997). Structural factor analyses for medically unexplained somatic symptoms of somatization disorder in the Epidemiologic Catchment Area study. *Psychological Medicine, 27,* 617–626.

Lloyd, A. R., Hickie, I., Brockman, A., Hickie, C., Wilson, A., Dwyer, J., et al. (1993). Immunologic and psychologic therapy for patients with chronic fatigue syndrome: A double-blind, placebo-controlled trial. *American Journal of Medicine, 94,* 197–203.

Lloyd, A. R., & Pender, H. (1992). The economic impact of chronic fatigue syndrome. *Medical Journal of Australia, 157,* 599.

Locke, G. R., III, Weaver, A. L., Melton, L. J., III, & Talley, N. J. (2004). Psychosocial factors are linked to functional gastrointestinal disorders: A population based nested case-control study. *American Journal of Gastroenterology, 99,* 350–357.

Looper, K. J., & Kirmayer, L. J. (2001). Hypochondriacal concerns in a community population. *Psychological Medicine, 31,* 577–584.

Lundh, L. G., & Simonsson-Sarnecki, M. (2001). Alexithymia, emotion and somatic complaints. *Journal of Personality, 69,* 483–510.

Lynch, P. M., & Zamble, E. (1989). A controlled behavioral treatment study of irritable bowel syndrome. *Behavior Therapy, 20,* 509–523.

Mai, F. M., & Merskey, H. (1980). Briquet's treatise on hysteria. A synopsis and commentary. *Archives of General Psychiatry, 37,* 1401–1405.

Martin, L., Nutting, A., Macintosh, B. R., Edworthy, S. M., Butterwick, D., & Cook, J. (1996). An exercise program in the treatment of fibromyalgia. *Journal of Rheumatology, 23,* 1050–1053.

Martin, R. (1991). Somatoform disorders in the general hospital setting. In F. K. Judd, G. D. Burrows, & D. R. Lipsitt (Eds.), *Handbook of studies on general hospital psychiatry* (pp. 251–265). New York: Elsevier.

Mayer, E. A., Naliboff, B., & Chang, L. (2001). Basic pathophysiologic mechanisms in irritable bowel syndrome. *Digestive Diseases, 19,* 212–218.

Mayer, E. A., Naliboff, B., & Munakata, J. (2000). The evolving neurobiology of gut feelings. *Progress in Brain Research, 122,* 195–206.

McCain, G. A., Bell, D. A., Mai, F. M., & Halliday, P. D. (1988). A controlled study of the effects of a supervised cardiovascular fitness training program on the manifestations of primary fibromyalgia. *Arthritis and Rheumatism, 31,* 1135–1141.

McCauley, J., Kern, D. E., Kolodner, K., Dill, L., Schroeder, A. F., DeChant, H. K., Ryden, J., et al. (1997). Clinical characteristics of women with a history of childhood abuse: Unhealed wounds. *Journal of the American Medical Association, 277,* 1362–1368.

McCrady, B. S., Stout, R., Noel, N., Abrams, D., & Nelson, H. (1991). Comparative effectiveness of three types of spouse involved alcohol treatment: Outcomes 18 months after treatment. *British Journal of Addictions, 86,* 1415–1424.

McEwen, B. S. (2005). Stressed or stressed out: What is the difference? *Journal of Psychiatry and Neuroscience, 30,* 315–318.

McHorney, C. A., Ware, J. E., Lu, J. F. L., & Sherbourne, C. D. (1994). The MOS 36–Item Short-Form Health Survey: III. Tests of data quality, scaling assumptions, and reliability across diverse patient groups. *Medical Care, 32,* 40–66.

McLeod, C. C., Budd, M. A., & McClelland, D. C. (1997). Treatment of somatization in primary care. *General Hospital Psychiatry, 19,* 251–258.

Mechanic, D. (1962). The concept of illness behavior. *Journal of Chronic Diseases, 15,* 189–194.

Mengshoel, A. M., Komnaes, H. B., & Forre, O. (1992). The effects of 20 weeks of physical fitness training in female patients with fibromyalgia. *Clinical and Experimental Rheumatology, 10,* 345–349.

Mennin, D. S., Heimberg, R. G., Turk, C. L., & Fresco, D. M. (2002). Applying an emotion regulation framework to integrative approaches to generalized anxiety disorder. *Clinical Psychology: Science and Practice, 9,* 85–90.

Meuret, A. E., Wilhelm, F. H., Ritz, T., & Roth, W. T. (2003). Breathing training for treating panic disorder: Useful intervention or impediment? *Behavior Modification, 27,* 731–754.

Minor, M. A. (1991). Physical activity and management of arthritis. *Annals of Behavioral Medicine, 13,* 117–124.

Moldofsky, H., & England, R. S. (1975). Facilitation of somatosensory average-evoked potentials in hysterical anaesthesia and pain. *Archives of General Psychiatry, 32,* 193–197.

Moldofsky, H., Lue, F. A., Mously, C., Roth-Schechter, B., & Reynolds, W. J. (1996). The effect of zolpidem in patients with fibromyalgia: A dose ranging, double blind, placebo controlled, modified crossover study. *Journal of Rheumatology, 23,* 529–533.

Moreno, J. L. (1975). Notes on the concept of role playing. *Group Psychotherapy and Psychodrama, 28,* 105–107.

Morin, C. M. (1993). *Insomnia: Psychological assessment and management.* New York: Guilford Press.

Morris, J. S., Ohman, A., & Dolan, R. J. (1999). A subcortical pathway to the right amygdala mediating "unseen" fear. *Proceedings of the National Academy of Sciences, 96,* 1680–1685.

Morriss, R. K., Wearden, A. J., & Battersby, L. (1997). The relation of sleep difficulties to fatigue, mood and disability in chronic fatigue syndrome. *Journal of Psychosomatic Research, 42,* 597–605.

Muller, T., Mannel, M., Murck, H., & Rahlfs, V. W. (2004). Treatment of somatoform disorders with St. John's wort: A randomized, double-blind and placebo-controlled trial. *Psychosomatic Medicine, 66,* 538–547.

Murphy, G. E. (1982). The clinical management of hysteria. *Journal of the American Medical Association, 247,* 2559–2564.

Mushin, J., & Levy, R. (1974). Averaged evoked responses in patients with psychogenic pain. *Psychological Medicine, 4,* 19–27.

Neff, D. F., & Blanchard, E. B. (1987). A multi-component treatment for irritable bowel syndrome. *Behavior Therapy, 18,* 70–83.

Nemiah, J. C., Freyberger, H., & Sifneos, P. E. (1976). Alexithymia: A view of the psychosomatic process. In O. W. Hill (Ed.), *Modern trends in psychosomatic medicine* (pp. 430–439). London: Butterworths.

Neria, Y., & Koenen, K. C. (2003) Do combat stress reaction and posttraumatic stress disorder relate to physical health and adverse health practices?: An 18-year follow-up of Israeli war veterans. *Anxiety, Stress and Coping, 16,* 227–239.

Newman, M. G., Castonguay, L. G., Borkovec, T. D., & Molnar, C. (2004). Integrative psychotherapy. In R. G. Heimberg, C. L. Turk, & D. S. Mennin (Eds.), *Generalized anxiety disorder: Advances in research and practice* (pp. 320–350). New York: Guilford Press.

Newton, T. L., & Contrada, R. J. (1992). Repressive coping and verbal-autonomic response dissociation: The influence of social context. *Journal of Personality and Social Psychology, 62,* 159–167.

Nicassio, P. M., Radojevic, V., Weisman, M. H., Schuman, C., Kim, J., Schoenfeld-Smith, K., et al. (1997). A comparison of behavioral and educational interventions for fibromyalgia. *Journal of Rheumatology, 24,* 2000–2007.

Nicassio, P. M., Schuman, C., Radojevic, V., & Weisman, M. H. (1999). Helplessness as a mediator of health status in fibromyalgia. *Cognitive Therapy and Research, 23,* 181–196.

Norcross, J. C. (2002). Empirically supported therapy relationships. In J. C. Norcross (Ed.), *Psychotherapy relationships that work: Therapist contributions and responsiveness to patients* (pp. 3–16). London: Oxford University Press.

Noyes, R., Langbehn, D. R., Happel, R. L., Stout, L. R., Muller, B. A., & Longley, S. L. (2001). Personality dysfunction among somatizing patients. *Psychosomatics, 42,* 320–329.

Offord, D. R., Boyle, M. H., Szatmari, P., Rae-Grant, N. I., Links, P. S., Cadman, D. T., et al.. (1987). Ontario Child Health Study, II: Six-month prevalence of disorder and rates of service utilization. *Archives of General Psychiatry, 44,* 832–836.

O'Leary, A. (1990). Stress, emotion, and human immune function. *Psychological Bulletin, 108,* 363–382.

O'Malley, P. G., Balden, E., Tomkins, G., Santoro, J., Kroenke, K., & Jackson, J. L. (2000). Treatment of fibromyalgia with antidepressants: A meta-analysis. *Journal of General Internal Medicine, 15,* 659–666.

Othmer, E., & DeSouza, C. A. (1985). A screening test for somatization disorder (hysteria). *American Journal of Psychiatry, 142,* 1146–1149.

Palsson, O. S., Turner, M. J., Johnson, D. A., Burnett, C. K., & Whitehead, W. E. (2002). Hypnosis treatment for severe irritable bowel syndrome: Investigation of mechanism and effects on symptoms. *Digestive Diseases and Sciences, 47,* 2605–2614.

Pappagallo, M. (2003). Newer antiepileptic drugs: Possible uses in the treatment of neuropathic pain and migraine. *Clinical Therapeutics, 25,* 2506–2538.

Parker, G., Cheah, Y. C., & Roy, K. (2001). Do the Chinese somatize depression?: A cross-cultural study. *Social Psychiatry and Psychiatric Epidemiology, 36,* 287–293.

Parker, G., Gladstone, G. L., & Chee, K. T. (2001). Depression in the planet's largest ethnic group: The Chinese. *American Journal of Psychiatry, 158,* 857–864.

Parsons, T. (1951). Illness and the role of the physician: A sociological perspective. *American Journal of Orthopsychiatry, 21,* 452–460.

Parsons, T. (1975). The sick role and the role of the physician reconsidered. *Milbank Memorial Fund Quarterly, 53,* 257–278.

Payne, A., & Blanchard, E. B. (1994). A controlled comparison of cognitive therapy and self-help support groups in the treatment of irritable bowel syndrome. *Journal of Consulting and Clinical Psychology, 63,* 779–786.

Perley, M. J., & Guze, S. B. (1962). Hysteria—the stability and usefulness of clinical criteria. *New England Journal of Medicine, 266,* 421–426.

Perls, F. (1973). *The Gestalt approach and eyewitness to therapy.* Palo Alto, CA: Science and Behavior Books.

Perquin, C. W., Hazebroek-Kampschreur, A. A., Hunfeld, J. A., Bohnen, A. M., van Suijlekom-Smit, L. W., Passchier, J., et al. (2000). Pain in children and adolescents: A common experience. *Pain, 87,* 51–58.

Persons, J. B. (1989). *Cognitive therapy in practice: A case formulation approach.* New York: Norton.

Peveler, R., Kilkenny, L., & Kinmonth A. L. (1997). Medically unexplained physical symptoms in primary care: A comparison of self-report screening questionnaires and clinical opinion. *Journal of Psychosomatic Research, 42,* 245–252.

Pilowsky, I. (1967). Dimensions of hypochondriasis. *British Journal of Psychiatry, 113,* 89–93.

Pilowsky, I. (1969). Abnormal illness behaviour. *British Journal of Medical Psychology, 42,* 347–351.

Powell, P., Bentall, R. P., Nye, F. J., & Edwards, R. H. T. (2001). Randomised controlled trial of patient education to encourage graded exercise in chronic fatigue syndrome. *British Medical Journal, 322,* 387–390.

Prins, J. B., Bleijenberg, G., Bazelmans, E., Elving, L. D., de Boo, T. M., Severens, J. L., et al. (2001). Cognitive behaviour therapy for chronic fatigue syndrome: A multicentre randomized controlled trial. *Lancet, 357,* 841–847.

Purtell, J. J., Robins, E., & Cohen, M. E. (1951). Observations on clinical aspects of hysteria: A quantitative study of 50 hysteria patients and 156 control subjects. *Journal of the American Medical Association, 146,* 902–909.

Quijada-Carrera, J., Valenzuela-Castano, A., Povedano-Gomez, J., Fernandez-Rodriguez, A., Hernanz-Mediano, W., Gutierrez-Rubio, A., et al. (1996). Comparison of tenoxicam and bromazepan in the treatment of fibromyalgia: A randomized, double-blind, placebo-controlled trial. *Pain, 65,* 221–225.

Radloff, L. S. (1977). The CES-D Scale: A self-report depression scale for research in the general population. *Applied Psychological Measurement, 1,* 1–24.

Rainville, J., Sobel, J., Hartigan, C., & Wright, A. (1997). The effect of compensation involvement on the reporting of pain and disability by patients referred for rehabilitation of chronic low back pain. *Spine, 22,* 2016–2024.

Raphael, K. G., Widom, C. S., & Lange, G. (2001). Childhood victimization and pain in adulthood: A prospective investigation. *Pain, 92,* 283–293.

Reik, T. (1948). *Listening with the third ear: The inner experience of a psychoanalyst.* New York: Grove Press.

Restak, R., Leong, S. A., Barghout, V., Birnbaum, H. G., Thibeault, C. E., Ben-Hamadi, R., et al. (2003). The economic consequences of irritable bowel syndrome: A U.S. employer perspective. *Archives of Internal Medicine, 163,* 929–935.

Reyes, M., Nisenbaum, R., Hoaglin, D. C., Unger, E. R., Emmons, C., Randall, B., et al. (2003). Prevalence and incidence of chronic fatigue syndrome in Wichita, Kansas. *Archives of Internal Medicine, 163,* 1530–1536.

Richards, S. C., & Scott, D. L. (2002). Prescribed exercise in people with fibromyalgia: Parallel group randomised controlled trial. *British Medical Journal, 325,* 185–189.

Rief, W., Heuser, J., Mayrhuber, E., Stelzer, I., Hiller, W., & Fichter, M. M. (1996).

The classification of multiple somatic symptoms. *Journal of Nervous and Mental Disease, 184,* 680–687.

Rief, W., & Hiller, W. (2003). A new approach to the assessment of the treatment effects of somatoform disorders. *Psychosomatics, 44,* 492–498.

Rief, W., Hiller, W., Geissner, E., & Fichter, M. M. (1995). A two-year follow-up study of patients with somatoform disorders. *Psychosomatics, 36,* 376–386.

Rief, W., Hiller, W., & Heuser, J. (1997). *SOMS—Screening fur Somatoforme Storungen. Manual Zum Fragebogen* [SOMS—Screening for Somatoform Symptoms—Manual]. Berne, Switzerland: Huber.

Rief, W., Hiller, W., & Margraf, J. (1998). Cognitive aspects of hypochondriasis and the somatization syndrome. *Journal of Abnormal Psychology, 107,* 587–595.

Rief, W., Shaw, R., & Fichter, M. M. (1998). Elevated levels of psychophysiological arousal and cortisol in patients with somatization syndrome. *Psychosomatic Medicine, 60,* 198–203.

Robins, L. N., Helzer, J. E., Croughan, J., & Ratcliff, K. S. (1981). National Institute of Mental Health Diagnostic Interview Schedule: Its history, characteristics, and validity. *Archives of General Psychiatry, 38,* 381–389.

Robins, L. N., & Reiger, D. (1991). *Psychiatric disorders in America: The Epidemiologic Catchment Area study.* New York: Free Press.

Robins, P. M., Smith, S. M., Glutting, J. J., & Bishop, C. T. (2005). A randomized controlled trial of a cognitive-behavioral family intervention for pediatric recurrent abdominal pain. *Journal of Pediatric Psychology, 30,* 397–408.

Robinson, D. N. (1996). *Wild beasts and idle humours: The insanity defense from antiquity to the present.* Cambridge, MA: Harvard University Press.

Roemer, L., & Orsillo, S. M. (2002). Expanding our conceptualization of and treatment for generalized anxiety disorder: Integrating mindfulness/acceptance-based approaches with existing cognitive-behavioral models. *Clinical Psychology: Science and Practice, 9,* 54–68.

Rogers, C. R. (1961). *On becoming a person.* Boston: Houghton Mifflin.

Roizenblatt, S., Moldofsky, H., Benedito-Silva, A. A., & Tufik, S. (2001). Alpha sleep characteristics in fibromyalgia. *Arthritis and Rheumatism, 44,* 222–230.

Rosanoff, A. J. (1938). *Manual of psychiatry and mental hygiene.* New York: Wiley.

Rose, S. D. (1977). *Group therapy: A behavioral approach.* Englewood Cliffs, NJ: Prentice Hall.

Rost, K., Kashner, T. M., & Smith, G. R. (1994). Effectiveness of psychiatric intervention with somatization disorder patients: Improved outcomes at reduced costs. *General Hospital Psychiatry, 16,* 381–387.

Rotunda, R. J., & O'Farrell, T. J. (1997). Marital and family therapy of alcohol use disorders: Bridging the gap between research and practice. *Professional Psychology: Research and Practice, 28,* 246–252.

Russo, J., Katon, W., Sullivan, M., Clark, M., & Buchwald, D. (1994). Severity of somatization and its relationship to psychiatric disorders and personality. *Psychosomatics, 35,* 546–556.

Salkovskis, P. M., & Warwick, H. M. C. (2001). Meaning, misinterpretations, and medicine: A cognitive-behavioral approach to understanding health anxiety and hypochondriasis. In V. Starcevic & D. R. Lipsitt (Eds.), *Hypochondriasis: Modern perspectives on an ancient malady* (pp. 202–222). New York: Oxford University Press.

Samoilov, A., & Goldfried, M. R. (2000). Role of emotion in cognitive-behavior therapy. *Clinical Psychology: Science and Practice, 7,* 373–385.

Sanders, M. R., Rebgetz, M., Morrison, M., Bor, W., Gordon, A,, Dadds, M., et al. (1989). Cognitive-behavioral treatment of recurrent nonspecific abdominal pain in children: An analysis of generalization, maintenance, and side effects. *Journal of Consulting and Clinical Psychology, 57,* 294–300.

Sanders, M. R., Shepherd, R. W., Cleghorn, G., & Woolford, H. (1994). The treatment of recurrent abdominal pain in children: A controlled comparison of cognitive-behavioral family intervention and standard pediatric care. *Journal of Consulting and Clinical Psychology, 62,* 306–314.

Sayar, K., & Ak, Y. (2001). The predictors of somatization: A review. *Bulletin of Clinical Psychopharmacology, 11,* 266–271.

Schofferman, J., & Wasserman, S. (1994). Successful treatment of low back pain and neck pain after a motor vehicle accident despite litigation. *Spine, 19,* 1007–1010.

Semler, G., Wittchen, H. U., Joschke, K., Zaudig, M., von Geiso, T., Kaiser, S., et al. (1987). Test–retest reliability of a standardized psychiatric interview (DIS/CIDI). *European Archives of Psychiatry and Clinical Neuroscience, 236,* 214–222.

Sharpe, M., Hawton, K., Simkin, S., Surawy, C., Hackmann, A., Klimes, I., et al. (1996). Cognitive behaviour therapy for the chronic fatigue syndrome: A randomised controlled trial. *British Medical Journal, 312,* 22–26.

Shaw, G., Srivastava, E. D., Sadlier, M., Swann, P., James, J. Y., & Rhodes, J. (1991). Stress management for irritable bowel syndrome: A controlled trial. *Digestion, 50,* 36–42.

Shorter, E. (1997). *A history of psychiatry: From the era of the asylum to the age of prozac.* New York: Wiley.

Siegel, D., Janeway, D., & Baum, J. (1998). Fibromyalgia syndrome in children and adolescents: Clinical features at presentation and status at follow-up. *Pediatrics, 101*(3), 377–382.

Sifneos, P. E. (1973). The prevalence of "alexithymic" characteristics in psychosomatic patients. *Psychotherapy and Psychosomatics, 22,* 255–262.

Simon, G. E., & Gureje, O. (1999). Stability of somatization disorder and somatization symptoms among primary care patients. *Archives of General Psychiatry, 56,* 90–95.

Simon, G. E., & Von Korff, M. (1991). Somatization and psychiatric disorder in the NIMH Epidemiologic Catchment Area Study. *American Journal of Psychiatry, 148,* 1494–1500.

Simon, G. E., & Von Korff, M. (1995). Recall of psychiatric history in cross-sectional surveys: Implications for epidemiologic research. *Epidemiological Review, 17,* 221–227.

Simon, G. E., Von Korff, M., Piccinelli, M., Fullerton, C., & Ormel, J. (1999). An international study of the relation between somatic symptoms and depression. *New England Journal of Medicine, 341,* 1329–1335.

Smith, G. R., & Brown, F. W. (1990). Screening indexes in DSM-III-R somatization disorder. *General Hospital Psychiatry, 12,* 148–152.

Smith, G. R., Monson, R. A., & Ray, D. C. (1986a). Patients with multiple unexplained symptoms: Their characteristics, functional health, and health care utilization. *Archives of Internal Medicine, 146,* 69–72.

Smith, G. R., Monson, R. A., & Ray, D. C. (1986b). Psychiatric consultation letter in somatization disorder. *New England Journal of Medicine, 314,* 1407–1413.

Smith, G. R., Rost, K., & Kashner, M. (1995). A trial of the effect of a standardized psychiatric consultation on health outcomes and costs in somatizing patients. *Archives of General Psychiatry, 52,* 238–243.

Smith, R. C., Gardiner, J., C., Lyles, J. S., Sirbu, C., Dwamena, F. C., Hodges, A., et al. (2005). Exploration of DSM-IV criteria in primary care patients with medically unexplained symptoms. *Psychosomatic Medicine, 67,* 123–129.

Soetekouw, P. M., de Vries, M., van Bergen, L., Galama, J. M., Keyser, A., Bleijenberg, G., et al. (2000). Somatic hypotheses of war syndromes. *European Journal of Clinical Investigation, 30,* 630–641.

Sonino, N., Navarrini, C., Ruini, C., Ottolini, F., Paoletta, A., Fallo, F., et al. (2004). Persistent psychological distress in patients treated for endocrine disease. *Psychotherapy and Psychosomatics, 73,* 78–83.

Speckens, A. E., Spinhoven, P., Sloekers, P. P., Bolk, J. H., & van Hemert, A. M. (1996). A validation study of the Whitely Index, the Illness Attitude Scales, and the Somatosensory Amplification Scale in general medical and general practice patients. *Journal of Psychosomatic Research, 40,* 95–104.

Speckens, A. E., van Hemert, A. M., Spinhoven, P., Hawton, K. E., Bolk, J. H., & Rooijmans, H. G. (1995). Cognitive behavioural therapy for medically unexplained physical symptoms: A randomized controlled trial. *British Medical Journal, 311,* 1328–1332.

Spielberger, C., Gorusch, R., & Lushene, R. (1970). *STAI manual.* Palo Alto, CA: Consulting Psychologists Press.

Spitzer, R. L. (1983). Psychiatric diagnoses: Are clinicians still necessary? *Comprehensive Psychiatry, 24,* 399–411.

Spitzer, R. L., Kroenke, K., & Williams, J. B. (1999). Validation and utility of a self-report version of PRIME-ID: The PHQ Primary Care Study. *Journal of the American Medical Association, 282,* 1737–1744.

Stekel, W. (1924). *Peculiarities of behaviour* (Vols. 1–2). London: Williams and Norgate.

Stevens, J. O. (1971). *Awareness: Exploring, experimenting, experiencing.* Lafayette, CA: Real People Press.

Stulemeijer, M., de Jong, L. W., Fiselier, T. J., Hoogveld, S. W., & Bleijenberg, G. (2005). Cognitive behaviour therapy for adolescents with chronic fatigue syndrome: Randomised controlled trial. *British Medical Journal, 330 (7481),* 14.

Sumathipala, A., Hewege, R., Hanwella, R., & Mann, A. H. (2000). Randomized controlled trial of cognitive behaviour therapy for repeated consultations for medically unexplained complaints: A feasibility study in Sri Lanka. *Psychological Medicine, 30,* 747–757.

Surawy, C., Hackmann, A., Hawton, K., & Sharpe, M. (1995). Chronic fatigue syndrome: A cognitive approach. *Behaviour Research and Therapy, 33,* 535–544.

Svedlund, J., Sjodin, I., Ottosson, J. O., & Dotevall, G. (1983). Controlled study of psychotherapy in irritable bowel syndrome. *Lancet, 2,* 589–592.

Swartz, M., Blazer, D., George, L., & Landerman, R. (1986). Somatization disorder in a community population. *American Journal of Psychiatry, 143,* 1403–1408.

Swartz, M., Hughes, D., George, L., Blazer, D., Landermann, R., & Bucholz, K. (1986). Developing a screening index for community studies of somatization disorder. *Journal of Psychiatric Research, 20,* 335–343.

Swartz, M., Landermann, R., George, L., Blazer, D., & Escobar, J. (1991). Somatization. In L. N. Robins & D. Reiger (Eds.), *Psychiatric disorders in America* (pp. 220–257). New York: Free Press.

Szasz, T. S. (1987). *Insanity.* New York: Wiley.

Takata, Y. (2001). Research on psychosomatic complaints by senior high school students in Tokyo and their related factors. *Psychiatry and Clinical Neurosciences, 55,* 3–11.

Talley, N. J. (2003). Evaluation of drug treatment in irritable bowel syndrome. *British Journal of Clinical Pharmacology, 56,* 362–369.

Talley, N. J. (2004). Antidepressants in IBS: Are we deluding ourselves? *American Journal of Gastroenterology, 99,* 921–923.

Talley, N. J., Boyce, P. M., & Jones, M. (1998). Is the association between irritable bowel syndrome and abuse explained by neuroticism?: A population-based study. *Gut, 42,* 47–53.

Taylor, G. J., Bagby, R. M., & Parker, J. D. A. (1997). *Disorders of affect regulation: Alexithymia in medical and psychiatric illness.* Cambridge, MA: Cambridge University Press.

Taylor, G. J., Bagby, R. M., Ryan, D. P., & Parker, J. D. (1990). Validation of the alexithymia construct: A measurement-based approach. *Canadian Journal of Psychiatry—Revue Canadienne de Psychiatrie, 35,* 290–297.

Taylor, R. R., & Leonard. J. A. (2001). Sexual abuse, physical abuse, chronic fatigue, and chronic fatigue syndrome: A community-based study. *Journal of Nervous and Mental Disease, 189,* 709–715.

Taylor, S. E., Klein, L. C., Lewis, B. P., Gruenewald, T. L., Gurung, R. A., & Updegraff, J. A. (2000). Biobehavioral responses to stress in females: Tend-and-befriend, not fight-or-flight. *Psychological Review, 107,* 411–429.

Teasdale, J. D. (1983). Negative thinking in depression: Cause, effect or reciprocal relationship? *Advances in Behavioural Research and Therapy, 5,* 3–25.

Thieme, K., Gromnica-Ihle, E., & Flor, H. (2003). Operant behavioral treatment of fibromyalgia: A controlled study. *Arthritis Care and Research, 49,* 314–320.

Thompson, W. G., Dotevall, G., Drossman, D. A., Heaton, K. W., & Kruis, W. (1989). Irritable bowel syndrome: Guidelines for the diagnosis. *Gastroenterology International, 2,* 92–95.

Thompson, W. G., & Heaton, K. W. (1980). Functional bowel disorders in apparently healthy people. *Gastroenterology, 79,* 283–288.

Thumboo, J., Fong, K. Y., Ng, T. P., Leong, K. H., Feng, P. H., Thio, S. T., et al. (1999). Validation of the MOS SF-36 for quality of life assessment of patients with systemic lupus erythematosus in Singapore. *Journal of Rheumatology, 26,* 97–102.

Todaro, J. F., Shen, B. J., Niaura, R., Spiro, A., Ward, K., & Weiss, S. (2003). A prospective study of negative emotions and CHD incidence: The normative aging study. *American Journal of Cardiology, 92,* 901–906.

Tofferi, J. K., Jackson, J. L., & O'Malley, P. G. (2004). Treatment of fibromyalgia with cyclobenzaprine: A meta-analysis. *Arthritis and Rheumatism, 51,* 9–13.

Tomasson, K., Kent, D., & Coryell, W. (1991). Somatization and conversion disorders: Comorbidity and demographics at presentation. *Acta Psychiatrica Scandinavica, 84,* 288–293.

Toner, B. B., Koyama, E., Garfinkel, P. E., & Jeejeebhoy, K. N. (1992). Social desirability and irritable bowel syndrome. *International Journal of Psychiatry in Medicine, 22,* 99–103.

Tsoi, W. F. (1985). Mental health in Singapore and its relation to Chinese culture. In W. Tseng & D. Wu (Eds.), *Chinese culture and mental health* (pp. 229–250). Orlando, FL: Academic Press Inc.

Ung, E. K., & Lee, D. S.-W. (1999). Thin desires and fat realities. *Singapore Medical Journal, 40,* 495–497.

Valdes, M., Garcia, L., Treserra, J., de Pablo, J., & de Flores, T. (1989). Psychogenic pain and depressive disorders: An empirical study. *Journal of Affective Disorders, 16,* 21–25.

Van Dulmen, A. M., Fennis, J. F., & Bleijenberg, G. (1996). Cognitive-behavioral group therapy for irritable bowel syndrome: Effects and long-term follow-up. *Psychosomatic Medicine, 58,* 508–514.

Veale, D., Kavanagh, G., Fielding, J. F., & Fitzgerald, O. (1991). Primary fibromyalgia and the irritable bowel syndrome: Different expressions of a common pathogenetic process. *British Journal of Rheumatology, 30,* 220–222.

Visser, S., & Bouman, T. K. (2001). The treatment of hypochondriasis: Exposure plus response prevention vs cognitive therapy. *Behaviour Research and Therapy, 39,* 423–442.

Vlaeyen, J. W., Teeken-Gruben, N. J., Goossens, M. E., Rutten-van Molken, M. P., Pelt, R. A., van Eek, H., et al. (1996). Cognitive-educational treatment of fibromyalgia: A randomized clinical trial. I. Clinical effects. *Journal of Rheumatology, 23,* 1237–1245.

Vollmer, A., & Blanchard, E. B. (1998). Controlled comparison of individual versus group cognitive therapy for irritable bowel syndrome. *Behavior Therapy, 29,* 19–33.

Volz, H. P., Moller, H. J., Reimann, I., & Stoll, K. D. (2000). Opipramol for the treatment of somatoform disorders results from a placebo-controlled trial. *European Neuropsychopharmacology, 10,* 211–217.

Volz, H. P., Murck, H., Kasper, S., & Moller, H. J. (2002). St John's wort extract (LI 160) in somatoform disorders: Results of a placebo-controlled trial. *Psychopharmacology, 164,* 294–300.

von Knorring, L., & Almay, B. G. (1989). Neuroendocrine responses to fen-fluramine in patients with idiopathic pain syndromes. *Nordisk Psykiatrisk Tidsskrift, 43,* 61–65.

von Knorring, L., Almay, B. G., Johansson, F., & Terenius, L. (1979). Endorphins in CSF of chronic pain patients, in relation to augmenting-reducing response in visual averaged evoked response. *Neuropsychobiology, 5,* 322–326.

Walker, E. A., Gelfand, A. N., Gelfand, M. D., & Katon, W. J. (1995). Psychiatric diagnoses, sexual and physical victimization, and disability in patients with irritable bowel syndrome or inflammatory bowel disease. *Psychological Medicine, 25,* 1259–1267.

Walker, E. A., Keegan, D., Gardner, G., Sullivan, M., Bernstein, D., & Katon, W. J. (1997). Psychosocial factors in fibromyalgia compared with rheumatoid arthritis: II. Sexual, physical, and emotional abuse and neglect. *Psychosomatic Medicine, 59,* 572–577.

Walker, L. S., Garber, J., & Greene, J. W. (1991). Somatization symptoms in pediatric abdominal pain patients: Relation to chronicity of abdominal pain and parent somatization. *Journal of Abnormal Child Psychology, 19,* 379–394.

Walker, L. S., Lipani, T. A., Greene, J. W., Caines, K., Stutts, J., Polk, D. B., et al. (2004). Recurrent abdominal pain: Symptom subtypes based on the Rome II criteria for pediatric functional gastrointestinal disorders. *Journal of Pediatric Gastroenterology and Nutrition, 38,* 187–191.

Waller, E., & Scheidt, C. E. (2006). Somatoform disorders as disorders of affect regulation: A development perspective. *International Review of Psychiatry, 18,* 13–24.

Ware, J. E., & Kosinski, M. (1996). *The SF-36 Health Survey (Version 2.0) Technical Note.* Boston: Health Assessment Lab.

Ware, J. E., & Sherbourne, C. D. (1992). The MOS 36–item short-form health survey (SF-36). *Medical Care, 30,* 473–483.

Ware, N. C. (1993). Society, mind and body in chronic fatigue syndrome: An anthropological view. In G. R. Bock & G. Whelan (Eds.), *Chronic fatigue syndrome* (pp. 62–82). Chichester, UK: Wiley.

Warwick, H. M., Clark, D. M., Cobb, A. M., & Salkovskis, P. M. (1996). A controlled trial of cognitive-behavioural treatment of hypochondriasis. *British Journal of Psychiatry, 169*(2), 189–195.

Wearden, A. J., Morris, R. K., Mullis, R., Strickland, P. L., Pearson, D. J., Appleby, L., et al. (1998). Randomized, double-blind, placebo-controlled treatment trial of fluoxetine and graded exercise for chronic fatigue syndrome. *British Journal of Psychiatry, 172,* 485–490.

Weissman, M. M., Myers, J. K., & Harding, P. S. (1978). Psychiatric disorders in a U.S. urban community: 1975–1976. *American Journal of Psychiatry, 135,* 459–462.

Welgan, P., Meshkinpour, H., & Beeler, M. (1988). Effect of anger on colon motor and myoelectric activity in irritable bowel syndrome. *Gastroenterology, 94,* 1150–1156.

Welgan, P., Meshkinpour, H., & Hoehler, F. (1985). The effect of stress on colon motor and electrical activity in irritable bowel syndrome. *Psychosomatic Medicine, 47,* 139–149.

Wessely, S., Chadler, T., Hirsch, S., Wallace, P., & Wright, D. (1997). The epidemiology of chronic fatigue and chronic fatigue syndrome: A prospective primary care study. *American Journal of Public Health, 87,* 1449–1455.

Wessely, S., Nimnuan, C., & Sharpe, M. (1999). Functional somatic syndromes: One or many? *Lancet, 354,* 936–939.

West, L. J. (1982). Introduction: Arthur Mirsky and the Evolution of Behavioral Medicine. In L. J. West & M. Stein (Eds.), *Critical issues in behavioral medicine* (pp. 59–69). Philadelphia: Lippincott.

Westen, D. (2000). Commentary: Implicit and emotional processes in cognitive-behavior therapy. *Clinical Psychology: Science and Practice, 7,* 386–390.

Weyerer, S., & Kupfer, B. (1994). Physical exercise and psychological health. *Sports Medicine, 17,* 108–116.

Whalen, P. J., Kagan, J., Cook, R. G., Davis, F. C., Kim, H., Polis, S., et al. (2004). Human amygdala responsivity to masked fearful eye whites. *Science, 306,* 2061.

Whalen, P. J., Rauch, S. L., Etcoff, N. L., McInerney, S. C., Lee, M. B., & Jenike, M. A. (1998). Masked presentations of emotional facial expressions modulate amygdala activity without explicit knowledge. *Journal of Neuroscience, 181,* 411–418.

White, G. M. (1982). The role of cultural explanations in "somatization" and "psychologization." *Social Science and Medicine, 16,* 1519–1530.

Whitehead, W. E., Crowell, M. D., Robinson, J. C., Heller, B. R., & Schuster, M. M. (1992). Effects of stressful life events on bowel symptoms: Subjects with irritable bowel syndrome compared with subjects without bowel dysfunction. *Gut, 33,* 825–830.

Whiting, P., Bagnall, A. M., Sowden, A. J., Cornell, J. E., Mulrow, C. D., & Ramirez, G. (2001). Interventions for the treatment and management of chronic fatigue syndrome: A systematic review. *Journal of the American Medical Association, 286,* 1360–1368.

Whorwell, P. J., Prior, A., & Faragher, E. B. (1984). Controlled trial of hypnotherapy in the treatment of severe refractory irritable bowel syndrome. *Lancet, 2,* 1232–1234.

Williams, D. A., Cary, M. A., Groner, K. H., Chaplin, W., Glazer, L. J., Rodriguez, A. M., et al. (2002). Improving physical functional status in patients with fibromyalgia: A brief cognitive behavioral intervention. *Journal of Rheumatology, 29,* 1280–1286.

Winkielman, P., & Berridge, K. C. (2004). Unconscious emotion. *Current Directions in Psychological Science, 13,* 120–123.

Wittchen, H. U. (1994). Reliability and validity studies of the WHO-Composite International Diagnostic Interview (CIDI): A critical review. *Journal of Psychiatric Research, 28,* 57–84.

Wolfe, F., Anderson, J., Harkness, D., Bennett, R. M., Caro, X. J., Goldenberg, D. L., et al. (1997). Work and disability status of persons with fibromyalgia. *Journal of Rheumatology, 24,* 1171–1178.

Wolfe, F., Ross, K., Anderson, J., Russell, I. J., & Hebert, L. (1995). The prevalence and characteristics of fibromyalgia in the general population. *Arthritis and Rheumatism, 38,* 19–28.

Wolfe, F., Smythe, H. A., Yunus, M. B., Bennett, R. M., Bombardier, C., Goldenberg, D. L., et al. (1990). The American College of Rheumatology 1990 criteria for the classification of fibromyalgia: Report of the Multicenter Criteria Committee. *Arthritis and Rheumatism, 33,* 160–172.

Wolpe, J. (1958). *Psychotherapy by reciprocal inhibition.* Stanford, CA: Stanford University Press.

Woodruff, R. A., Jr., Clayton, P. J., & Guze, S. B. (1971). Hysteria: Studies of diagnosis, outcome, and prevalence. *Journal of the American Medical Association, 215,* 425–428.

Wool, C. A., & Barsky, A. J. (1994). Do women somatize more than men?: Gender differences in somatization. *Psychosomatics, 35,* 445–452.

Woolfolk, R. L. (1998). *The cure of souls: Science, values, and psychotherapy.* San Francisco: Jossey-Bass.

Woolfolk, R. L., Allen, L. A., Gara, M. A., & Escobar, J. I. (1998). *The Somatic Symptom Questionnaire.* Unpublished manuscript.

Woolfolk, R. L., & Lehrer, P. M. (Eds.). (1984). *Principles and practice of stress management.* New York: Guilford Press.

World Health Organization. (1979). *The ICD-9 classification of mental and behavioural disorders: Diagnostic criteria for research.* Geneva, Switzerland: Author.

World Health Organization. (1993). *The ICD-10 classification of mental and behavioural disorders: Diagnostic criteria for research.* Geneva, Switzerland: Author.

World Health Organization. (1994a). *Composite international diagnostic interview (CIDI).* Washington, DC: American Psychiatric Press.

World Health Organization. (1994b). *Schedules for clinical assessment in neuropsychiatry (SCAN).* Washington, DC: American Psychiatric Press.

World Health Organization. (1994c). *Somatoform disorders schedule.* Geneva, Switzerland: Author.

Yehuda, R. (1997). Sensitization of the hypothalamic-pituitary-adrenal axis in posttraumatic stress disorder. *Annals of the New York Academy of Sciences, 821,* 57–75.

Yehuda, R., Golier, J. A., Halligan, S. L., Meaney, M., & Bierer, L. M. (2004). The ACTH response to dexamethasone in PTSD. *American Journal of Psychiatry 161,* 1397–1403.

Yunus, M. B., Masi, A. T., & Aldag, J. C. (1989a). A controlled study of primary fibromyalgia syndrome: Clinical features and association with other functional syndromes. *Journal of Rheumatology, 16* (Suppl. 19), 62–71.

Yunus, M. B., Masi, A. T., & Aldag, J. C. (1989b). Short-term effects of ibuprofen in primary fibromyalgia syndrome: A double-blind placebo controlled trial. *Journal of Rheumatology, 16,* 527–532.

Yutzy, S. H., Cloninger, R., Guze, S. B., Pribor, E. F., Martin, R. L., Kathol, R. G., et al. (1995). DSM-IV field trial: Testing a new proposal for somatization disorder. *American Journal of Psychiatry, 152,* 97–101.

Zajonc, R. B. (1980). Feeling and thinking: Preferences need no inferences. *American Psychologist, 35,* 151–175.

Zhang, W. X., Shen, Y. C., & Li, S. R. (1998). Epidemiological investigation on mental disorders in seven areas of China. *Chinese Journal of Psychiatry, 31,* 69–71.

Zoccolillo, M., & Cloninger, C. R. (1986). Somatization disorder: Psychologic symptoms, social disability, and diagnosis. *Comprehensive Psychiatry, 27,* 65–73.

Zung, W. W. (1965). A self-rating depression scale. *Archives of General Psychiatry, 12,* 63–70.

Zwaigenbaum, L., Szatmari, P., Boyle, M. H., & Offord, D. R. (1999). Highly somatizing young adolescents and the risk of depression. *Pediatrics, 103,* 1203–1209.

Index

Abbreviated progressive muscle relaxation
  diaphramatic breathing and, 96
  instructions for, 187–188
  overview, 96, 98–99
  10-session treatment manual and, 160
Abdominal breathing. *See* Diaphramatic
  breathing
Abnormal illness behavior, 30–34. *See also*
  Illness behaviors
Abridged somatization
  impact of on healthcare system, 30–31
  overview, 24–25
  See also Subthreshold somatization
Abuse history
  clinical presentation of somatization and,
    32–34
  comorbidity and, 146–147
Activities, increasing
  overview, 99–102
  significant other, involvement of in
    treatment and, 136–137
  10-session treatment manual and, 156, 161
Activity pacing
  overview, 103–104
  10-session treatment manual and, 156
Adolescents, somatization in, 44–45
Adreno-medullary response, 48
Affect, labeling of, 110–111. *See also* Emotion
Affective cognitive-behavioral therapy
  assertiveness training and, 133
  behavioral management and, 99–109
  clinical trial assessing efficacy of, 165–172,
    169*t*, 170*f*, 171*f*
  cognitive restructuring and, 126–129
  emotional awareness training and, 110–111,
    112*f*, 113–115, 116*t*, 119–124, 141–142
  group therapy and, 147–150
  overview, 85–86, 86–91

  rationale for, 63–65, 87–90, 154
  relationships with healthcare providers, 91–
    93
  relaxation training and, 95–99
  10-session treatment manual for, 85–86, 153–
    164
  therapeutic relationship and, 93–94
Alexithymia, 53–54
Allostatic load, 50
Alosetron, 35–36
Amitriptyline, 36
Amplification, somatosensory, 82–83
Anti-inflammatories, 35
Anticholinergic/antispasmodic agents, 35
Anticonvulsants, 142
Antidepressants
  overview, 142–143
  treatment outcome research on, 34–35
Antiepileptic agents, 35
Anxiety disorders
  comorbidity with, 29, 31–32, 146–147
  pharmacological interventions and, 142–143
  somatic symptoms and, 29
Appraisals
  cognition, behavior and social learning
    theory, 58–59
  cognitive restructuring techniques and, 126–
    129
Assertiveness training
  overview, 133–135
  10-session treatment manual and, 162
Assessment
  clinical interview, 69–72, 72–74
  in clinical practice, 66–72, 83–84
  in clinical trial assessing efficacy of affective
    cognitive-behavioral therapy, 167–168
  cognitive and behavioral disturbances, 82–
    83

219